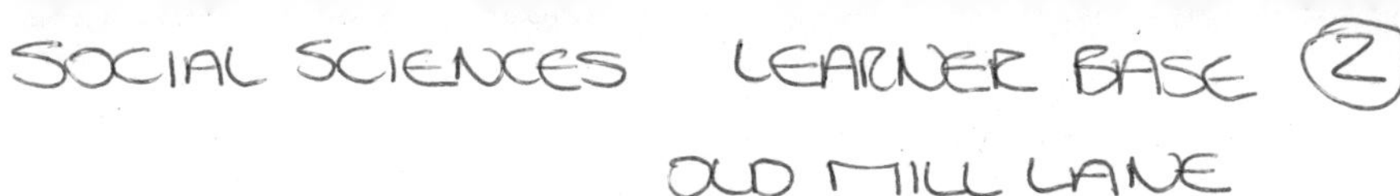

Worlds of illness

The burden of illness is having to live with it in the world of the healthy.

In recent years the study of illness as experienced by patients has emerged as an approach to understanding sickness and health. Descriptions of the everyday situations of people with particular diseases provide a commentary upon the nature of symptoms and upon the relation of the body to society. This approach stresses the biographical and cultural contexts in which illness arises and is borne by individuals and those who care for them. It emphasizes the need to understand illness in terms of the patient's own interpretation, of its onset, the course of its progress and the potential of the treatment for the condition.

Worlds of Illness examines people's experience of illness and their understanding of what it means to be healthy. It brings together, for the first time in one volume, contributors from a variety of fields who use a biographic and cultural approach. They define the biographical/cultural perspective further and draw attention to its potential for questioning theoretical assumptions about sickness and health. *Worlds of Illness* is important as a contribution to ongoing debates in medical sociology, and to developments in health psychology which has recently emerged as an active research field.

Alan Radley is Senior Lecturer in Social Psychology at Loughborough University.

Worlds of illness

Biographical and cultural perspectives on health and disease

Edited by Alan Radley

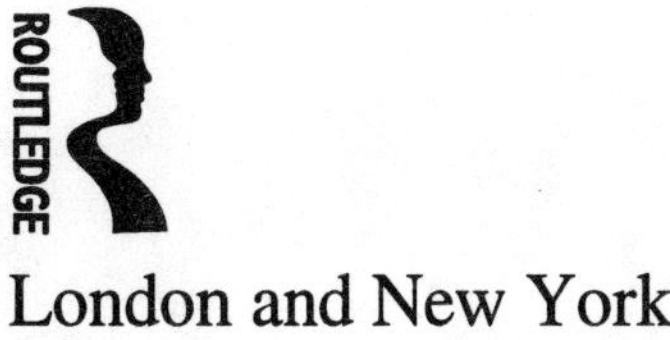

London and New York

For Marg, belatedly

First published in 1993
by Routledge
11 New Fetter Lane, London EC4P 4EE

Simultaneously published in the USA and Canada
by Routledge
29 West 35th Street, New York, NY 10001

First published in paperback 1995

Typeset in Times New Roman by Michael Mepham, Frome, Somerset
Printed and bound in Great Britain
by Mackays of Chatham PLC

A Tavistock/Routledge Publication

British Library Cataloguing in Publication Data
A catalogue record for this book is available from the British Library

Library of Congress Cataloguing in Publication Data
A catalogue record for this book is available from the
Library of Congress

ISBN 0-415-06769-3 (hbk)
ISBN 0-415-13152-9 (pbk)

Contents

Figures and tables

FIGURES

TABLES

Contributors

Paul Bellaby is Senior Lecturer in Sociology and Director of the Centre for Health Policy Research at the School of Economic and Social Studies, University of East Anglia. Formerly at the University of Keele, he is author of *The Sociology of Comprehensive Schooling* together with numerous articles on adolescence and social control in schools, the occupational strategies of nurses, sickness absence and work organization and risk and culture.

Alan Blair is currently working as a clinical psychologist in North Derbyshire in adult community mental health and is conducting research into the organizational dynamics of occupational stress in health service employees. He is also an Honorary Research Fellow at the University of Birmingham. In addition to his research into the role of social class in the experience and expression of distress, he has researched extensively in the area of eating behaviour. He has also written a number of critical reviews of clinical psychology interventions in specific areas, most recently on work carried out in the field of primary prevention.

Mildred Blaxter is Honorary Professor of Sociology at the School of Economic and Social Studies, University of East Anglia. Research interests have included disability and chronic illness, lay concepts of health, the health of children, the measurement of health, social and behavioural aspects of HIV/AIDS, and inequalities. Publications include *The Meaning of Disability* (1976); *The Health of the Children* (1981); *Mothers and Daughters* (with E. Paterson), (1982); *Health and Lifestyles* (1990); *AIDS: Worldwide Policies and Problems* (1991).

Tom Kitwood is a senior lecturer in social psychology at Bradford University, and Director of Bradford Dementia Research Group. His recent work has been concerned with opening up a field that might be termed 'the social psychology of senile dementia', and with the promotion of good practice in dementia care. Before this his research focussed mainly on psychological aspects of ethics, values and moral development. His publications here include *Disclosures to a Stranger* (1981) and *Concern for Others* (1991).

Martha MacLeod is Project Adviser Nursing, St. Boniface General Hospital, and Adjunct Professor in the Faculty of Nursing, University of Manitoba, Winnipeg, Canada. Currently, she is planning and teaching in collaborative undergraduate and post-graduate nursing courses. Her research concerns the everyday experience of students, nurses and surgical patients, and how people learn in the midst of their everyday experience. She writes about nursing practice and learning, and serves on the editorial boards of the Journal of Nursing Education and the Journal of Clinical Nursing.

Janine Pierret is a sociologist at the Centre de Recherche Médecine, Maladie et Science Sociales (CERMES-CNRS) in Paris, where she is a Director of Research. Her special area of interest is the effect of chronic illness upon family and professional life. Recently, she has been comparing the everyday life patterns and identity changes of groups of AIDS sufferers with different histories – hemophiliacs, heterosexuals and homosexuals. She is the author, with Claudine Herzlich, of *Illness and Self in Society*, (1987) *Malades d'hier, malades d'aujourdhui*, (1991).

Kristian Pollock studied social anthropology at Edinburgh University before carrying out postgraduate research into popular concepts of health and illness in Britain. Particular interests include the use of knowledge and ideas about illness as a 'resource' in the adaptation of sufferers and their families to serious mental and physical disorder, and the use (and abuse) of 'stress' as an explanation for such misfortune. Since completing her thesis at Cambridge University in 1984 she has combined bringing up four children with part–time work for the Open University.

Alan Radley is Senior Lecturer in Social Psychology in the Department of Social Sciences at Loughborough University, U.K. His research in the area of health and illness has centered upon the social and psychological adjustment of coronary patients and their families to bypass graft surgery. He is also concerned with the development of theory concerning the place of the body in social life. He is the author of *Prospects of Heart Surgery: psychological adjustment to coronary bypass grafting*, (1988); *The Body and Social Psychology*, (1991); and co-author of *Ideological Dilemmas: a social psychology of everyday thinking*, (1988).

Gareth Williams is Senior Research Fellow in Sociology of Health and Illness in the Centre for Health Studies at University College Salford, and the Department of Sociology at the University of Salford. He has written on the subjects of chronic illness and disability for both medical and sociological journals and is co-editor (with Stephen Platt, Sue Scott, and Hilary Thomas) of *Private Risks and Public Dangers* (1991) and *Locating Health: Historical and Sociological Explorations* (1992). He is currently involved in research projects on lay perspectives on health, health care, and the urban environment, and the specification and implementation of contracts in the area of community health services.

Rory Williams is currently Senior Research Scientist at the Medical Research Council's Medical Sociology Unit at Glasgow University. His present research interests are in the connection of ethnicity and religion with health, and with the economic factors which affect health. These interests arise out of work on the economic and religious background in attitudes to death and illness. He is the author of *A Protestant legacy: attitudes to death and illness among older Aberdonians* (1990).

Acknowledgements

This book was put together with the aid of 'new technology'. This, however, means organizing contributions written in different formats and using different software packages. I am deeply grateful to Mavis Hearnden of the Computer Centre at Loughborough University who translated the software, and to Jo Wakefield of the Department of Social Sciences who helped to re-format the disks where necessary. Without their help the novelty of the technology would certainly have worn off, and this book been slower in its production.

Introduction

Alan Radley

Over the past twenty years the study of illness as experienced by patients has emerged as an approach to understanding sickness and health in general. From descriptions of the everyday situations of people with particular diseases, a commentary has been made upon the nature of symptoms and upon the relation of the body to society. This approach stresses the biographical and the cultural contexts in which illness arises and is borne by patients and those who care for them. It emphasizes the need to understand illness in terms of the patient's own interpretation of its onset, the course of its progress and the potential of the treatment for the condition.

Underlying the application of this approach is the claim that many important questions about illness – in which context it arises, what action is taken to seek treatment, its effects on other areas of life – need to be asked in the light of how people comprehend it as part of their own life situation.

The emphasis upon biographical understanding is consistent with the need to study illness in its cultural context. In this case, how people make sense of and respond to their disease or disability is a function of the everyday beliefs and practices attaching to their social groupings. These in turn are shaped by the ideologies of illness produced in society by the efforts of doctors and others to secure a cure for these conditions.

This approach makes illness something more than a temporary break in an otherwise healthy existence. This is partly the result of many present-day ailments being relatively chronic diseases, with which people have to live as best they can (Anderson and Bury 1988). The prevalence of complaints such as heart disease, multiple sclerosis and rheumatoid arthritis tend to figure the illness condition, while at the same time reflecting other aspects of life through its intrusions and the ways with which these are dealt. This is one reason why the world of illness is not separated from the sphere of health, as might be thought when focusing upon temporary, acute afflictions only.

However, it is not just the kinds of problem that researchers choose to study which determine the form of their inquiries. There has arisen a broad theoretical orientation that understands illness as something that people not only suffer, but as a condition that can call for a re-negotiation of their social identity (Gerhardt 1989). This results from the fact that there is a stigmatizing element to illness, in response to which individuals must strive, not only to surmount their difficulties, but to do so in ways that are socially acceptable and appropriate.

There is, therefore, a problem of how to manage one's illness; there is also the problem of the resources with which one can make the required adjustments. The first is a question of ways of coping, of the means whereby people work out their response to illness and their passage through its course. The second problem relates to the social positioning of individuals, to differences and inequalities and more particularly to ideologies and practices that are associated with medical diagnosis and treatment. In both cases there is often more than a little borrowing from the various domains of health in the person's construction of what might be called an 'illness-world'.

This approach to understanding illness has begun to highlight the taken-for-granted assumptions concerning the question of health, and what people regard as the necessary conditions for leading a healthy lifestyle and for avoiding disease (Blaxter 1990). In recent years there has emerged a concern to understand how people conceptualize health and illness, so that the relationship between these terms is placed in question (Herzlich 1973). Such research not only tells us how people think of health and what causes it to be breached; it also tells us about the assumptions (or social representations) that articulate people's experience of the sick and of their own periods of illness. Therefore, the worlds of illness and of health cannot be wholly separate because they inform each other; how this happens has important implications for theory and for methodology in this field of research.

This collection of essays contributes to this stream of inquiry. Although the papers draw upon a variety of contexts to illustrate work in their various fields, each one offers ideas that resonate about a number of themes. One of these is the theme of health itself, considered as an inquiry into the interpretive system underlying people's views about how one stays healthy or falls ill (Pierret). There is an important sense in which health 'is not just a value but an event which people can use to interpret their relations with the social order'. The challenge to sociology is to understand how the discourses that appear to attach only to issues of health and illness also help to construct the relationship of the individual to society.

This analysis of the lay perspective shows that how people think about health and illness varies with their position in society, so that this discourse is itself informed by their interests in other spheres of life. One aspect of social difference is position in the production system, where the specific cultural practices in which people are enjoined and their means of expressing these, will locate their experience of illness in a specific context. Examining the linguistic resources available for conceptualizing suffering reveals that there are important differences in the way that people from different social backgrounds formulate illness (Blair).

The finding that middle-class people tend to view illness in mentalistic terms, while individuals from working-class backgrounds are more likely to see it in physicalist terms has implications for how patients orientate themselves towards therapy and recovery. It also has implications for the kinds of moral judgements that are made about the sick, by themselves and by others. These judgements have been shown to vary according to the disease in question, with varying degrees of personal responsibility being accorded to those suffering from what are seen as either physical or mental disorders. In trying to cope with physical disease it is often believed that what is important is an attitude of mind that involves fighting the illness, not giving in to adversity. What becomes clear is that this strategy, although having various degrees of success, often does not square with the reality of the condition. In spite of this, the belief in self-help can provide a 'rhetoric of optimism', though at the same time being the basis of the charge that failure to cope is the result of either a 'defective or inadequate will' (Pollock).

This double-sidedness of the ideology of coping shows that the study of health beliefs has not merely revealed that different sections of the population hold different views about a variety of diseases. One important strand in this work has been the discovery of ambiguities and contradictions in the way that people talk about health and disease (see also Rogers 1991). Evidence that people may 'borrow' discourses and practices from other sources in order to make sense of their illness situation calls for finer-grained analyses than have been carried out so far (Pierret).

An example of this borrowing is provided by appeal to one source of meaning that has received relatively little attention in the literature of medical sociology to date – religion. A study of religion in this context provides more than another survey of a resource that people can use in times of distress. It also introduces questions about the place of cosmologies that serve to structure personal beliefs about 'the powers of the individual versus those of society, and both versus the involuntary powers of the body and the natural world' (Rory Williams). If we are to understand how illness and health are conceived, then the fact that religious beliefs accommodate the notion of death is surely sufficient reason for including them in future research.

The focus upon social representations of health and illness is consistent with another theme of the book; how the sick cope with their illness and how they are expected to do so by others. The idea that illness in particular faces individuals with moral imperatives is revealed in the accounts given by those who must cope with chronic illnesses of one kind or another. The world of illness is shown to be one that involves not just a functional adjustment, but what is called here the 'pursuit of virtue' (Gareth Williams). The attempt by sick individuals to show their position as legitimate and themselves as worthy derives from views in society (which they often share) about the need for independence and for self-affirmation. Living with a disabling disease is shown to be an ongoing expression of the validity of one's life, through the (more or less) successful articulation of mundane acts which are thereby rendered as moral practices. This reinforces once more the idea that the experience of health and illness is not reducible to the level of individual motive: ways of being well and of bearing illness are instances and embodiments of ideology and social practice.

Chronic illness, in particular, faces people with the prospect of living with a disease, of having to adjust in some way to a life rendered different. There is, however, no universal response to suffering, in spite of the fact that people share beliefs about illness with others. One reason for this, as mentioned above, is that individuals have access to different resources in society, including means of linguistic expression. Another reason is that there is a wide variation in what might be called the domains of everyday experience, so that what must be made sense of during sickness will vary considerably. The double need of the sick to legitimate their position and to render inchoate experience tangible is discussed here in terms of metaphor (Radley). For the chronically sick who must live with illness in a world of health, the continuing attempts at resolving the contradictory demands of others sometimes result in a particular use of figurative language. Such metaphor serves not only to link different domains of experience (to 'borrow' in Pierret's terms), and to grasp the metaphysical (in Rory Williams's terms) but to pose the individual as worthy in the attempt to meet these difficult demands.

One potential outcome of failure to account successfully for one's illness is to blame oneself for falling prey to the disease. This is interesting, given that those who are most exposed to health risks in their everyday lives are more likely to give behavioural or physicalist causes for falling ill. Addressing this question directly shows that, although people recognize the health deficits of a relatively deprived background, they also import these very deficits into their current self-descriptions, transforming weaknesses into strengths (Blaxter). Simplicity of lifestyle and hardship do not only constrain or weaken; for those who outlast these contingencies they are sources of pride, virtues in a world that values a robust attitude to issues of health.

To understand how these apparently contradictory views can co-exist, it is necessary to see them as part of a 'chain of cause'. What individuals say about their illness is given structure by their need to strive for some experiential coherence in their accounts. This emphasizes that expressed beliefs about health and illness are not merely sampled from a pre-existing system of socially shared thought, but are articulated accounts that serve more than one purpose. One of these purposes is the search for meaning, the need to render suffering and uncertainty tangible and, at least, subject to anticipation if not to prediction. Another purpose, as pointed out already, is to enable the afflicted person to appear a creditable and worthy individual. It appears that it is this that is placed at risk if one blames only one's environment; self-blame is shown, paradoxically, as one strand in the discourse of self-legitimation.

A less prominent, but by no means less important issue underlying the papers in this book is the relationship of the sick person to medical practitioners and to medical knowledge. The focus upon chronic illness that is in evidence in many of the chapters is not a fortuitous one. It arises from an approach which, in attempting to comprehend the illness experience within the biographical situation of the patient, breaches the division between the person and the disease. To speak of ways of coping or of adjustment implies a view of sickness that is beyond the boundaries set by the notion of the passive patient, who is at the hands of a doctor treating only what can be objectified. Two chapters illuminate the opposite ends of this spectrum with regard to the approach of medical staff. One shows how senile dementia continues to be conceptualized firmly within the biomedical approach, so that for many sufferers the consequence of this is to be labelled as being beyond hope (Kitwood). In contrast to the medical view, empirical support for which is questioned in this chapter, there have emerged other, subsidiary discourses. Among these is the attempt to recover the person from the disease category by the use of a biographical approach. The value of such an account in the present context is that it illustrates what can be at stake in the struggle to give space to the biographical and cultural context of disease. The very issues that have been described above – including the need to come to terms with 'the darkest fears that confront the human race' – are seen to be struggling for inclusion in the debate about the fate of elderly persons who are judged to be 'dementing'.

Senile dementia shares one special feature with a condition shown to be prevalent among young adults – closed head injury (Bellaby). Both involve a patient who lacks full consciousness of his or her condition, so that the work of adjustment to illness must be carried on by carers, who are often members of the immediate family. They are involved in reconstructing the disruption to the patient's biography in a way that must take due account of the 'liminal' position in which society places such individuals. The point is made that the prominence that medicine gives to adjustment by the (conscious) individual (i.e. its individualized approach) makes for difficulties where an important part of the recovery is initiated by others. The issues of 'proper' adjustment, however, remain; the difference is that these are also to be understood in terms of the legitimation of the carers' (e.g. family's) actions, in relation to the official moralities available (see also Voysey 1975).

These points about Alzheimer's Disease and closed head injury are part of a wider debate about the relationship of sick people to the institution of medicine. Although this volume does not take up these issues on a wide scale, it acknowledges that to speak about illness in a biographical context is to invite a re-thinking of the relationship of patients to health-care staff. The understanding of medical terminology by laypeople is something that has received more attention in the literature than the way that medical staff use cultural knowledge in their work. One chapter in this volume goes some way to remedying this imbalance, by questioning the assumption that nurses know their patients through formal knowledge, aggregates of separate perceptions and skills (MacLeod). Instead, it is argued that nurses come to know patients through an intersubjective practice. This is not an abstract or theoretic exercise, being grounded in the pragmatics of the work of the hospital; instead, this practice is reflected as a form of moral enterprise. The activities of nursing involve the care of bodies by touch and manipulation, so that patients' conceptions of illness are here reflected through a praxis that establishes their moral worth, not just defines their objective illness condition. The parallels between these nursing practices and ideas of care in severe chronic illness await disclosure within the kind of approach that can embrace concepts like health, self-worth and vulnerability within a single scheme. In the meanwhile, this contribution reminds us that the study of health and illness must include an analysis of the way in which people take up (or refuse) the dominant discourse in Western culture that defines these things as 'medical matters'.

There is a more general argument to be made on the basis of the material offered in these chapters. It illustrates the dangers of decontextualizing illness and its management, thus abstracting the individual from his or her social setting. By so doing one brackets out the circumstances that mediate illness, its causes, the resources available for coping, the scope for adjustment and for availing oneself of the health-care system. The presentation of chronic illness as a domain in which the person must strive to retain moral worth is jeopardized by a reduction of his or her situation to one of good 'self-care management' conducted upon the basis of value-free scientific principles.

The emphasis upon biography and cultural setting in these papers highlights the potential, and sometimes the limitations, of the patient to signify as an individual. At one level, this is revealed in the fact that this power is less available to members of those groups who, for economic and other reasons, already hold a secondary place in the social order. There are people (e.g. the 'dementing' elderly) who can be considered to be marginalized with respect to the main cultural assumptions about health care. It might be said that all people who suffer from chronic illnesses of one kind or another have their identities placed at risk. However, for these and other marginal groups the expression of their situation, the articulation of suffering and the means of complying with the dominant ideology about coping are more difficult because of the construction of their respective places within society. One point coming from a number of the papers presented here is that notions of 'healthy lifestyle' and 'good adjustment' are most readily granted to those individuals who are in a position to signify as persons of moral worth, and as free of blame for their condition. Elaborating this argument in future is one important contribution that can be made by the kind of approach illustrated in this book.

The chosen methodology for much of the work presented in the chapters is the qualitative interview. While research into chronic illness in medical sociology has not been noted for its methodological rigour (Bury 1991), several of the authors are explicit in their justification of the approach which they have taken in the collection of their data. The use of the interview as a tool of ethnography allows several aims to be achieved; it gives a first-hand report of the situation of the patient, his or her everyday life experience and social situation; it reveals how individuals re-present constructions about health and illness that are sensed by them as originating in society; it locates these issues in the complex of other life-concerns, from which reports of health status are often abstracted by other methods, and in consequence misappropriated; it allows for not only a 'designative' but also an 'expressive' (Gareth Williams) form of discourse in which the situated and temporal construction of knowledge is pre-supposed; and finally, the use of interview material can be reflected against survey data in order to refine and develop concepts put forward in previous publications.

These points add up to the conclusion that the study of people's worlds of health and of illness is not just a catalogue of individual experiences of disability, of despair or of victory over suffering. To see it only in this way is to oppose this research to the biomedical and empiricist tradition, in which illness is assumed to be the disruption of material bodies subject to an objective environment. The counterpart of this tradition, and its support, is the view that there are subjective experiences, in this context a 'patient's view', that needs to be accommodated also. By indicating the ways in which individual illness experience reflects the social order, and in taking it up reconstitutes it, the chapters that follow show the limitations of this subjectivist position.

It is one of the main aims of this volume to indicate the potential of this research area for posing new and worthwhile questions in social scientific study. If nothing else, this work focuses attention upon the body as a site, not only of moral ambiguity in everyday life, but of theoretical reconstruction in both sociological and in social psychological inquiry (Radley 1991; Turner 1984, 1987).

The above resumé weaves together a number of common threads in the papers to follow; the order of the chapters reflects the structure of this argument. However, each chapter is intended to stand alone as a report of work in the particular field chosen by the author concerned. Therefore, it is intended that readers will sample them in the order that fulfils their own particular interests. It is confidently hoped that, in doing this, they will derive wider benefits than those that could be anticipated from the brief summary given above.

REFERENCES

Anderson, R. and Bury, M. (eds) (1988) *Living with Chronic Illness: the experience of patients and their families*, London: Unwin Hyman.

Blaxter, M. (1990) *Health and Lifestyles*, London: Routledge.

Bury, M. (1991) 'The sociology of chronic illness: a review of research and prospects', *Sociology of Health and Illness* 13: 451–68.

Gerhardt, U. (1989) *Ideas about Illness: an intellectual and political history of medical sociology*, London: Macmillan.

Herzlich, C. (1973) *Health and Illness: a social–psychological analysis*, London: Academic Press.

Radley, A. (1991) *The Body and Social Psychology*, New York: Springer-Verlag.

Rogers, W.S. (1991) *Explaining Health and Illness: an exploration of diversity*, London: Harvester Wheatsheaf.

Turner, B.S. (1984) *The Body and Society*, Oxford: Blackwell.

Turner, B.S. (1987) *Medical Power and Social Knowledge*, London: Sage.

Voysey, M. (1975) *A Constant Burden: the reconstitution of family life*, London: Routledge & Kegan Paul.

1 Constructing discourses about health and their social determinants[1]

Janine Pierret

HEALTH AND ILLNESS IN SOCIOLOGY

For a long time, medical sociology has, from a Parsonian perspective, oriented research toward the themes of the sick role and illness behaviour. In the 1970s, its outlook broadened as Parsonian frames of reference were reappraised by Berkanovic (1972), Gallagher (1976), Gerson (1976), Gerhardt (1978) and Alonzo (1984). These and other scholars directed very pertinent criticisms at this way of seeing illness as 'deviance' and doctors as agents of social control. They pointed out that this model, having arisen out of the study of acute diseases, could not account for the present-day reality of chronic illness. They added that it does not treat ill persons like actors who work out their own conceptions of illness and have an active part in medical care as they cope with their condition. Furthermore, the Parsonian perspective overlooks topics such as prevention, the variety of health-care structures and the role of a patient's family and friends. It has also been alleged that this model is medicocentric, since it postulates the ill person's obligation to seek medical care, specifically allopathic medical treatment.

Within this context of critical reappraisal, analytical models were reworked so as to take into account not just the individual's relation to medicine and medical professionals but also the totality of his activities and relations with other actors (notably family members) concerned by the illness. Several studies of the illness experience and patients' subjective feelings were conducted in order to examine their adjustments to illness and management of everyday life (Strauss and Glaser 1975; Speedling 1982; Schneider and Conrad 1983; Radley and Green 1987; and Radley 1988).

Meanwhile, particularly in Europe, the social sciences were showing more interest in 'ordinary people', 'the patient's point of view' or the 'lay perspective'. Closer attention was being paid to the 'contents' of notions of illness and health and especially to beliefs about the 'cause of disease', which were taken to be cognitive bits of information. Although these beliefs do not furnish a coherent model, the way was thus opened for inquiry into the ill individual's sense of responsibility and vulnerability (Chrisman 1977; Helman 1978; Pill and Stott 1982; Blaxter 1983; D'Houtaud and Field 1984). Adopting a broader approach, Herzlich (1973) probed French middle-class 'social representations' of health and illness. Several other scholars also proposed lay classifications, or definitions, based on the 'structural' – economic or cultural – context (Blaxter and Paterson 1982; Williams 1981, 1983 and 1990; Cornwell 1984; Crawford 1984; and Calnan 1987). Most of this research was carried out in specific groups: usually among women, certain age-groups or the working classes. To enlarge upon these populations, Backett (1990) carried out research among middle-class women and men in Edinburgh, Scotland.

The theme of health itself has gradually come to the forefront of research. This is not, of course, unrelated to the emergence of health as a key value in Western civilization – to what Crawford (1980) has called a 'new health consciousness'. New notions, such as 'health behaviour' or 'health promotion', have made it possible to take into account 'life-styles'. At the same time, various measures have been devised; and there are now 'subjective' health indicators, like those used in the Nottingham Health Profile (Hunt and McEwen, 1980), of persons' attitudes and behaviours. Despite this research on indicators and on individuals' health behaviours, ambiguity persists: the forementioned notions are still often defined in terms, such as 'preventive behaviours' or 'behaviours for health' (Anderson *et al.* 1988), that are consistent with what medical professionals consider to be comportments that forestall, or retard, illness or accidents.

While this research was being conducted on individuals' behaviours, other studies, particularly in Great Britain, were focusing on the social determinants of health at the macrolevel. Light has thus been shed on inequalities between social groups, between the sexes and between generations, especially since publication of the Black Report (Townsend and Davidson 1982; Blaxter and Paterson 1982; Cornwell 1984; Calnan and Johnson 1985; and Calnan 1987). In her survey of this research, Macintyre (1986: 393) has preferred using the phrase 'social patterning' to refer to these differences in matters of health and reserving the term 'inequality' for the social class inequalities. Her objective was to correlate health, measured in various ways, with the variables of occupational class, gender, marital status, age, ethnic group and place of residence. Likewise, the Health and Life-Style Survey of 9,003 persons carried out from 1984 to 1985 in England, Wales and Scotland focused on behaviours, attitudes and inequalities related to health, its definition and distribution in the population:

The definition of health used in this study, therefore, is essentially multi-

> dimensional and relative. It includes both objective and subjective components, and attempts to consider the positive as well as the negative range.
>
> (Blaxter, 1990: 4)

As the sociology of health makes progress, several questions crop up. How do qualitative and quantitative approaches intersect? How can data gathered among individuals be used in the quest for an explanation at the macrolevel? How does the way information is gathered affect a person's talk about health? How to correlate personal behaviours and social determinants? Several social scientists have emphasized the need to link discourses and behavioural determinants, the micro-and macrolevels. This holds especially for those who, like Cornwell (1984) or Williams (1990), have gathered qualitative information through in-depth interviews, biographies and case studies about lay conceptions of health and illness. For Calnan (1987):

> One of the problems of adopting this kind of interpretive approach alone is that it cannot deal with, or is not concerned with, how, where and why ideas generate. Yet a comprehensive approach to health and illness should also be able to account for how and why and under what conditions certain rules and beliefs emerged and are sustained. Thus there is a need to adopt a frame of reference that can also show how perceptions about health and illness are shaped by structural and cultural elements.
>
> (Calnan 1987: 8)

HEALTH AS A SYSTEM OF INTERPRETATION

Sociology's tendency to focus on illness rather than health is related to the saliency of the biomedical viewpoint. But also, as Augé (1984), an anthropologist, has pointed out, it is illness that is 'eventful' in a person's life as well as in the evolution of a society. By revealing that bodies are not working right, illness serves as the basis for interpretations that bring social relations into play and under review. Hence, in Fainzang's (1989) words, health is on the side of social order and norms:

> Discourse about illness works like a grid for interpreting an individual's social relations; and in parallel, ideas about health ... are the subject of a discourse in intaglio wherein health is the absence of an impression made by others upon one self. ... To talk, or even think, about health would, therefore, be to think of one's self as pristinely innocent, freed from all social relations.
>
> (Fainzang 1989: 438–9)

I do not fully agree with this. On the contrary, I think health, like illness, is a topic of lay discourses, which can be analysed as systems of interpretation.

Sociologists have described the emergence of health as a value in terms of a 'new health and fitness consciousness', 'healthism' or the 'duty to be healthy' (Zola 1977; Crawford 1977 and 1980; Renaud 1981; and Herzlich and Pierret 1987). Although this 'bodyism' lays emphasis on self-development, pleasure and hedonism, it has also come along with a trend that makes individuals responsible for their health and thus cultivates a sense of discipline. Crawford (1984) has discerned two tendencies in American health consumerism:

> Self-control and release understood as resistance, like their function as cultural mandates, must be seen as two sides of the same coin. It is the same society that paradoxically makes it difficult for us to attain control over the conditions that shape our everyday lives while concurrently undermining our capacity for 'healthful' release from imposed and internalized controls.
>
> (Crawford 1984: 97)

For these two tendencies, health is not just a value but also, in Augé's words, an 'event', which people can use to interpret their relations with the social order.

Sociology must show how lay, or commonsense, discourses are constructs that enable individuals to understand and interpret social reality. Herzlich (1984b) has dwelled on this idea, shared by several sociologists, in her analysis of 'social representations':

> Through their analysis, researchers must try to link the fact that, far from being a reflection of reality, a social representation constructs this reality with the fact that this representation reaches beyond each individual and is partly presented to him as coming from somewhere else.
>
> (Herzlich 1984b: 77)

In his review of research on lay models of health and illness, Calnan (1985) has stated his position:

> The application of the social construction approach to health and illness focuses on the way sufferers make sense of their body and bodily disturbances. Emphasis is therefore placed on examining lay interpretive processes within the context of lay knowledge and beliefs. Thus, rather than treating health beliefs as idiosyncratic, this type of approach emphasizes their logic and integrity.
>
> (Calnan 1985: 90)

These constructs form systems – they are made up of interrelated elements organized through a unifying principle, rationale or logic. Thanks to these systems, individuals find a meaning in what is happening to them and find their bearings in society. In Fitzpatrick's (1984) words:

> Some anthropologists take seriously the term 'system' when they talk of a community's belief system with regard to health and illness. Essentially they argue that the beliefs about illness identified in a community should be analyzed in terms of a system in the sense that beliefs are held to be interconnected and structured elements of a whole, rather than a random set of items that a group of people happen to believe in common.
>
> (Fitzpatrick 1984: 19)

Moreover, belief systems are systems of interpretation. They are 'reservoirs of signs' to be used to construct reality and interpret how each person stands in relation to the social order. For Herzlich (1984a):

> The collective interpretation of illness is done by using terms that, strictly speaking, cast doubt on society or the social order. ... Because it requires an interpretation, illness conveys meaning: it becomes a significant with a signifié that is the individual's relation to the social order.
>
> (Herzlich 1984a: 202)

My interest in health aroused, I conducted a survey – independently of any connotations about medicine or disease – with the aim of understanding the lay meaning of health, which was, at the time, becoming a key value. My perspective was quite different from the one adopted in public health surveys (see WHO's definition of health; Stacey 1976 and Anderson 1984), which operationalize the notion of health. My interest in this notion necessitated a very broad perspective. Interviews seemed best suited for providing people with the chance to freely express feelings as they talk about their lives and practices. In fact, my objective was to go much deeper than the contents of lay definitions of health in order to discover, beyond the variety of these contents or definitions, the interpretive system underlying discourses. An additional objective was to use a qualitative and a quantitative approach so as to correlate constructs of health in these discourses with 'structural' elements.

THE SURVEY AND ITS METHODOLOGY

With these objectives in mind, I gathered both qualitative data through in-depth interviews and quantitative data through a closed questionnaire. This survey, conducted in 1980, covered 111 persons, who belonged to one of three subsamples: residents of an old quarter in Paris; residents of a 'new city' (built at 60 km from Paris); and farmers from a rural commune in southern France. The two urban subsamples, each of about 50 persons, were demographically and socioeconomically comparable.

Each interview started with the following broad, impersonal statement: 'I would like you to tell me about health, about what it means to you'. During exploratory interviews, the phrase 'your health' had been used, but it induced talk about illness. During the survey proper, persons were not, when appointments were set, clearly told about the theme, which was left in very general terms referring to life-ways but without alluding to illness or medicine. Nearly 200 hours of interviews were recorded and fully transcribed. This provided several thousand pages of data.

After each interview, a questionnaire with 77 questions was left behind. This questionnaire was intended for a systematic analysis of what, at the time, the French Public Health Administration called a 'global conception of health'. It inquired into several 'areas' of everyday life. Three sorts of information about interviewees could thus be gleaned: demographic and socioeconomic data; data about living conditions (housing, work, transportation), habits (food, tobacco and alcohol) and recourse to medical care (and the health system in general); and opinions about conditions related to jobs or the environment.

A content analysis revealed the various ways persons reacted when they were asked, at the start of the interview, about health. In addition, it provided a list of the themes spontaneously mentioned during interviews: work and life at work, food, housing, environment, illness, its causes, and the care provided for it by institutions, by family and friends and by interviewees themselves. Talk about health entailed telling about one's self and about others – about one's relations with others and with society. Interviewees thus had the opportunity to mention various practices and preoccupations. When analysing how talk was organized, I thought it worthwhile to focus on the speaker's stance and adoption of a 'register' for talking.[2] I hypothesized that the way an interviewee reacted from the start to the request to talk about health shaped what would be said during the rest of the interview. In other words, by the end of the first few minutes, he or she had adopted a register for organizing what would be said from then on. This adoption of a register was related to, first of all, the individual's type (personal or impersonal) of concern about health matters and, secondly, his or her general ideas about health. This bears a resemblance to Cornwell's (1984) procedure of noting the order in which points were mentioned so as to distinguish between 'private' and 'public accounts', the former being made at the start of the interview. However, I felt the register adopted at the start of the interview was more important than this difference between public and private accounts.

By observing the first words, phrases, questions or silences that followed my introduction, I discerned four registers, each corresponding to the interviewee's type of concern and general ideas about health. The following abridged phrases shall be used to refer to them:

a) 'Health-illness': In a personal way, these interviewees associated health with illness and medicine.
b) 'Health-tool': In an abstract, impersonal way, these interviewees thought that health had a value and was a form of wealth.
c) 'Health-product': In a personal way showing their concern, these interviewees took health to be an objective to be reached, but they thought that reaching it depended on several factors.
d) 'Health-institution': In a distant, impersonal way, these interviewees stated that health was a matter of public policy and institutions.

The interviews were then submitted to a cross-sectional analysis by theme. When asked to talk about health, all interviewees spontaneously talked about illness and care for it; and eight out of ten referred to work and careers. The third most frequently mentioned theme had to do with food consumption: food quality, kinds of produce and the organization of meals. One out of two interviewees dwelled on the theme of preventing illness and thus told about their physical activities as well as the consumption of tobacco and alcoholic beverages. One out of three said something about housing and the immediate environment. Obviously, asking people to tell me about health amounted to asking them to talk about their activities in general, their social environment and their relations with it. Each of the forementioned themes was analysed in order to verify the hypothesis about the four registers adopted from the start.

These interviews could then be used to reconstruct homogeneous discourses about health. Thanks to this reconstruction, I identified four autonomous, coherent ways interviewees organized their talk. Each of these constructs the discourse within its social setting and enable it to take on meaning. These ways of organizing talk about health into coherent discourses constitute the codes that individuals in the same society or group use to communicate, as Moscovici (1973), Herzlich (1984b) and Jodelet (1989) have pointed out about 'social representation'. These reconstructed discourses bring to light the systems used to interpret persons' relations to their environment.

CONSTRUCTING DISCOURSES ABOUT HEALTH

The forementioned idea of 'register' was not intended for analysing the contents of lay notions of health (for a full account of these contents, see Pierret 1984). In fact, as research in various lands has shown, these contents are relatively stable but contradictory. My intent was to see how the tensions, or contradictions, observed in discourses about health are resolved.

With this in mind, I could identify elements running through several themes: the importance given to personal experience, the individual's sense of time, his feeling of responsibility for his health, and his dual involvement in production and consumption. These elements, which organized talk into a discourse, refer to a 'moral universe' (or, we might say, a universe of moral discourse) where they take on meaning. In this universe, the discourse becomes coherent as tensions within it are resolved. It is this universe that makes it possible to interpret the individual's relation to the social order. After identifying contradictions in lay discourses about health, Williams proposed analysing the way in which such contradictions are worked out in practice, and the way they have been shaped in the first place by assumptions, doctrines and discourses about economy, society and religion.

(Williams 1990: 12)

Health-illness: health means not being sick

This register gave the feeling of the interviewee's personal experience of illness. In these interviews, talk was organized around the tension between 'not being sick' and 'being well'. This tension corresponds to what Herzlich (1973: 56 and 60) has called 'health-in-a-vacuum', which is simply the 'absence of illness', and health as a balance implying 'physical and psychological well-being'. In a broader sense, this tension sets an 'impersonal fact' at odds with a 'personal equilibrium' one is trying to reach (Herzlich 1973: 63). It could be heard in the type of argumentation used throughout the interview, regardless of the topic. This argumentation was binary: 'all or nothing' – 'You got it [health], or you don't'. It rang through the following oppositions: healthy/unhealthy, normal/pathological and moderate/excessive. For these interviewees, illness is an excess, which may make people aware of what is normal as they undergo the experience of restoring an equilibrium. This restoration calls for the help and knowledge of medical professionals, because illness is a sudden, unforeseeable event that makes one helpless.

In their research on nineteenth-century French proverbs about the body, Loux and Richard (1978) have shown how very important moderation was. They thus brought to light a lay theory about respecting the equilibrium – order – of the universe. A cycle, rhythm or 'natural history' were key ideas in this construct of health, whose unifying principle seemed to be a certain conception of time. This order, or equilibrium, had to be respected since every event followed a 'natural cycle' and one could never make up for what had passed. According to Stacey (1986: 14), this positive conception of health as an equilibrium is more frequently found in French than British studies.

This construct of health is organized around the tension between the absence of illness and a state of physical and mental well-being. In the moral universe where this tension is resolved, 'the order of things' and 'the golden mean' reign. This order corresponds to a 'normal life', a phrase not necessarily implying fatality or determinism. It is this specific moral universe to which interpretations of the individual's relations with others and with society are referred.

Health-tool: when you got health, you got everything

Some interviewees talked in an impersonal, general way and presented health as 'what's most important'. For them, health was the principal form of wealth: with it, everything became possible, in particular work. This construct was shaped by the tension between possessing this form of wealth (avoir la santé: having health) and using health as a tool (in order 'to be able to work').

Health is a capital that everyone has. As a biological characteristic of the individual, it corresponds to what Herzlich (1973: 58) has called a 'reserve of health' associated with the person's 'constitution' and 'resistance'. Health has value; it is the mainstay of a life rhyming with work. This sort of capital is inherited at birth. This 'gift of nature' must be 'kept up' since it wastes away over time. Hence, the individual must try to keep it from being worn down or, at least, to delay this inevitable wear-and-tear. In this way, one remains capable of coping with everyday life and bearing up under the burdensome constraints of work. However the individual is, ultimately, helpless against the inexorable passing of time.

Since illness is a 'fault', medical professionals will not be consulted until it is no longer possible to do without their help. Cornwell has commented on this moralistic conception:

> There are obvious reasons why work and health should be connected in people's minds. Illness can incapacitate and prevent people from working. In doing so, it can threaten not only the practical basis of their lives but also their moral reputation. The moral philosophical argument which connects the two is less obvious, but it is none the less fundamental to the recurrent theme in public accounts of health and illness – of 'good health' being a morally worthy state and illness being discreditable.
>
> (Cornwell 1984: 127)

From a different perspective, Dodier (1984), too, has shown how a moral universe is constructed for interrelating health and working conditions at the workplace. This conception of health might be likened to the theory of human capital developed by economists, such as Grossman (1972). Accordingly, health is a 'durable good' with which everyone is endowed at birth. Although it depreciates over time, it can be renewed through an 'investment' that combines various 'factors of production' – medical treatments or healthy behaviours for preventing illness.

On the other hand, health is a tool to be used on the job. Work is the reference mark for organizing all of life. This almost 'organic' link between health and work is part of a functional conception of health as the 'capacity for doing' things and as 'what is needed in order to do' things. These two aspects are visible in British research on working-class women and the elderly: health as the strength to resist illness and as the ability to cope with everyday demands (Blaxter and Paterson 1982; Pill and Stott 1982; Cornwell 1984; Calnan 1987; and Williams 1983). For Williams (1990: 50–1), 'constitutional strength' is a 'moral matter' which is 'something one must be at least partly responsible for' whereas 'incapacity for tasks' is a 'mechanical matter' 'exempt from responsibility or blame'. None the less, both these aspects 'fit into schemes of understanding which are complementary but opposed'.

There is a tension between ideas of health as an indispensable tool for work and as a capital with which one is endowed at birth (and which, therefore, is independent of one's will) but that time wears down. This tension is resolved by adopting an ethic of duty and endurance so as to cope with whatever fate one is dealt. For Williams (1990), the roots of this work ethic, observed among older residents in Aberdeen, ran back into economic history and the Protestant tradition. When a similar ethic of work and duty can be observed in a Catholic land like France, we are led to wonder whether it may be related to the economic model of nineteenth-century industrialization and capitalism. But will this ethic survive a permanently high rate of structural unemployment?

Health-product: it all depends on ...

Some interviewees talked in a very personal, concerned way about health being the outcome of a set of factors over which the individual had a large degree of control. For them, health was a personal value, the supreme reference mark. All of life was organized for health's sake.

This construct entails ongoing tension between: controllable and uncontrollable factors; the private and public spheres; living conditions and the social environment; a 'me-cult' and a relatively 'sensible' management of one's life; consumption and the exigencies of one's position in the production system; and finally, the exaltation of personal freedom and the demands of state and society. In brief, tension is generated by, on the one hand, the quest for pleasure and, on the other, the assessment and control of risks. For Crawford (1984: 94), the tension between what he has described as 'release' and 'self-control' is resolved through a 'new health consciousness' which belongs to neither control nor release. People often speak of the necessity for 'balance' or the avoidance of 'extremes'. And certainly, each symbol and its corresponding experiences find their power in opposition, an opposition that is perhaps basic to human life.

In my survey, interviewees resolved this tension by referring to a moral universe where pleasure rather than control or discipline reigns: 'Be happy!' This is what Bourdieu (1979: 409) has called the morals of the 'duty to have fun'.

Health-institution: health is a matter of policy

This register of discourse was distant and impersonal; and health was seen from a collective, political viewpoint. Health was health policy, which implied national and local programmes for preventing and treating illness. Health was not so much a private 'good' as a collective heritage, which society should manage by developing facilities and implementing a policy for reducing inequality. This discourse, which places health beyond the scope of personal, individual management, may call for imposing discipline on all citizens.

The tension shaping this discourse arises between the welfare state's beneficient interventions and its use of force. Installing collective facilities entails programming, or planning, which, in turn, may necessitate coercive or disciplinary measures. The moral universe for resolving this tension is the world of citizenship and 'social rights'.

Other studies have not found this health-institution construct. Is it peculiarly French? Does this moral universe have its origins in the centralizing, Jacobinic tradition? Or has it arisen out of the history of the welfare state and social policy in France alone?

The organizing dimensions of these discourses

These four health constructs provide several contrasts. As for the speaker's stance, it is personal in health-illness and health-product but impersonal and rather abstract in health-tool and health-institution. In the health-illness construct, health is a norm having to do with personal experiences and opinions; in the health-product construct, a personal value and a controllable factor; in the health-tool construct, an impersonal form of wealth; and in the health-institution construct, a collective, political heritage. Responsibility for health is: professional, medical and curative in the health-illness and health-tool constructs; individual and preventive in the health-product construct; and public and governmental in the health-institution construct. In the health-illness and health-tool constructs, time inevitably erodes health, wears down the body and menaces the individual whereas, in the health-product and health-institution constructs, life can be controlled and managed. In the health-illness and health-tool constructs, the individual's relation to the world of production and work is of key importance whereas the role as a consumer is what counts in the health-product and health-institution constructs.

Each of these ways of constructing a discourse is coherent and forms a system. Health as well as illness fit into these global systems of interpretation that situate the individual in society. The tensions shaping each of these constructs are resolved by the reference to a moral universe: the 'natural order' in the health-illness construct, the notion of duty in the health-tool construct, the idea of pleasure in the health-product construct, and the conception of citizenship in the health-institution one. Health turns out, as Fainzang (1989: 438) stated, to be a grid of interpretation that can be used to resolve certain contradictions arising out of social relations.

SOCIAL DETERMINANTS

Besides reconstructing these discourses and their organizing principles, I also inquired into the conditions wherein they are produced. With what social variables were these constructs correlated? Should these correlations be explained? By identifying the tensions in each discourse and their resolution in the corresponding moral universe, interrelations between health, illness and work had come to light. These interrelations could be observed not only in what each interviewee said about their own experience but also through a general, abstract discourse about collectively shared experiences. Williams (1990) has laid heavy emphasis on the meaning of the interrelation between work and health:

> Among the biographical experiences that shaped Aberdonians' ideas about coping, one of the most prominent was the meaning which they had found in their working life. Some aspects of this meaning were class specific ... much was more generally concerned with work as a moral value and as generational experience.
>
> (Williams 1990: 222)

To explain the interrelation between work and health, I chose to focus not on age but on the individual's position in the world of work.

As a first step, I sought out the most significant correlations between the social variables contained in the questionnaire and the forementioned constructs of health; but this statistical analysis yielded disappointing results. In particular, INSEE's socioeconomic classification, traditionally used in France, proved inadequate.[3] Given my sample's size, I could not use each variable as such, but had to combine them in order to localize interviewees' positions in the production system. Information about these variables now came from both the questionnaires (e. g., occupation and level of education) and interviews (e. g., job contents and characteristics). The following information was put to use: whether interviewees were working in the private or public sectors; whether or not they had stable employment with relative job security; and the nature and level of education and of job qualifications. Five groups were thus formed out of the interviewees who were working:

1 small farmers;
2 un-or semiskilled workers and persons with unstable jobs;
3 middle-level employees in the private sector;
4 middle-level employees in the public sector; and
5 secondary school teachers in public schools.

Each group comprised an equal number of men and women who were (a) less than 40 years old, and (b) over 40.

In this way, I reconstructed the grid of interpretation devised by each of these groups. These grids came out of and reflected interviewees' positions in the system of production (for more details, see Pierret 1988). For those with manual occupations (i.e., the first two groups), whose bodies were 'tools' or 'implements' used on the job, health was seen in relation to work as both the ability to cope and the absence of illness. For farmers, illness and risk fit into a relatively homogeneous world-view based on a cycle of life involving work, health and nature. They felt as though they exercised some control over their health. This did not hold for the workers and persons with unstable employment; they felt socially vulnerable. For them, illness, though unforeseeable, does inevitably wear the body down. The three other groups – more or less middle-class – had a certain level of education and worked in the tertiary sector in occupations requiring training or know-how. What discriminated between them was whether their jobs were in the private or public sectors, as we can see from their world-views. Health, not illness, was at the centre of their attention. When talking about health, the two public-sector groups referred to their conceptions of social order: middle-level employees emphasized social inequality in health matters; and teachers thought illness was a 'social problem' calling for a collective response. The middle-level private-sector employees had individual, hedonistic ideas about bargaining pleasure for health.

This analysis, based on groups empirically defined by their positions in the production system, shed light on systems of interpretation compatible with, though not identical to, the previously discussed constructs of discourses about health. How are these systems and constructs related?

For manual workers and small farmers, there were strong tensions between health, illness and work. As already pointed out, there were two sources of tension: not being sick vs. being well; and health as wealth vs. health as a tool. The moral universe serving as a reference for them was the 'order of things' as imposed by work, which was felt to be a duty. This corresponds to the health-illness and health-tool constructs. In order to understand non-manual employees' interpretations of work and of the social order, I had to take into account the value placed on health and the sector (public or private) where they worked. The middle-level private-sector employees were individualists who saw the world in terms of the pleasure/risk opposition. Since they tended to give more importance to pleasure, we discover something similar to the health-product construct. In contrast, public-sector wage-earners, whether middle-or upper-level, tended to see themselves as citizens; their understanding of health was collective and governmental. It corresponds to the health-institution construct.

In France, persons' relations to the State, in particular whether they work in the private or public sectors, seems to be as important as social class origins. This result differs from findings in Great Britain, in particular by Calnan (1987), who, although he contrasted the individualistic tendencies of the middle classes to the collectivist tendencies of the working class, added: 'However, this distinction ... presents an oversimplified picture; and many respondents from both social groups displayed ambivalence in their policies' (Calnan 1987: 93).

These results call for a finer, deeper analysis. For one thing, the means used to observe or measure social determinants need to be redesigned by replacing existing categories with new ones. For another, we might be able to find social determinants by focusing on factors other than the individual's position in the production system. We might, for example, focus on the type of housing, leisure activities or even food patterns, and thus define an indicator of a person's 'conditions of existence'.

In conclusion, the relations between the sociologist's construction and reconstruction of the same set of interviews are complex. The constructs based on the interviewee's adoption of register highlighted the way people talked, and what they felt, about health but left in the shadows the actual contents of their talk. When this same material was reworked as a function of the interviewee's position in the production system, the tension between health, illness and work – already brought to light through the forementioned constructs – turned out to be much more important.

Might discourses about health (and illness) be organized not as a function of the variables retained herein but on the basis of 'constants', such as a person's sense of time, relations to the State or feeling of security? Should we perhaps look for constants of this sort when trying to find the social determinants of discourses? Do individuals, depending on their positions in the production system, 'borrow', usually selectively, discourses and practices from other sources, past or present, in the society? Under what conditions does this borrowing occur, and to what end? Does it have to do with how material conditions affect the production of ideas? In any case, whether we are trying to construct social determinants or lay discourses about health, the latter, as they emerge out of interviews, are definitely social constructs that can be analysed as systems of interpretation. These systems reach far beyond the field of health and medicine. They are organized around logics, or rationales, involving: the person's sense of time, the private/public dimension of life at home and life on the job, and ideas of risk and security as well as of production and consumption.

NOTES

Translated from French by Noal Mellott, CNRS, Paris.

1 I would like to thank Claudine Herzlich for her careful reading of this text. Her perspicacious comments were helpful during the rewriting.
2 The term 'register' is not used in the linguistic sense herein.
3 Desrosières and Thévenot (1988) have criticized INSEE's socioeconomic categories (catégories socio-professionnelles, CSP). Since 1982, these have been reformulated as occupational and socioeconomic categories (professions et catégories socio-professionnelles, PCS). The major headings in this classifications are: 1. farmers; 2. craftsmen, merchants and businessmen; 3. upper-level white-collars and 'intellectual professions'; 4. middle-level occupations; 5. lower-level employees; and 6. workers.

REFERENCES

Alonzo, A.A. (1984) 'An illness behavior paradigm: a conceptual exploration of a situational-adaptation perspective', *Social Science of Medicine 19* (5): 499–510.
Anderson, R. (1984) 'Health promotion: An overview', *European Monographs in Health Education Research* 6: 4–119.
Anderson, R., Davies, J.K., Kickbusch, I., McQueen, D.V. and Turner, J. (1988) *Health Behaviour Research and Health Promotion*, Oxford University Press.
Augé, M. (1984) 'Ordre biologique, ordre social: la maladie forme élémentaire de l'événement', in Augé, M. and Herzlich, C. (eds) *Le sens du mal. Anthropologie, histoire, sociologie de la maladie*, Paris: Editions des Archives Contemporaines, 35–91, English translation forthcoming, *The meaning of illness*, Reading: Gordon and Breach.
Backett, K.C. (1990) 'Studying health in families: a qualitative approach', in

Cunningham-Burley, S. and McKeganey, N.J. (eds) *Readings in medical sociology*, London: Tavistock Publications.

Berkanovic, E. (1972) 'Lay Conceptions of the Sick Role', *Social Forces*, 51: 53–64.

Blaxter, M. (1983) 'The causes of disease: Women talking', *Social Science and Medicine* 17 (2): 58–69.

Blaxter, M. (1990) *Health and Lifestyles*, London: Routledge.

Blaxter, M. and Paterson, E. (1982) *Mothers and daughters: a three-generational study of health attitudes and behaviour*, London: Heinemann Educational Books.

Bourdieu, P. (1979) *La distinction: critique sociale du jugement*, Paris: Editions de Minuit.

Calnan, M. (1985) 'Lay interpretations and reponses to illness', in Morgan, M., Calnan M. and Manning, N. (eds) *Sociological Approaches to Health and Medicine*, London, Sydney: Croom Helm, 76–105.

Calnan, M. (1987) *Health and illness: the lay perspectives*, London: Tavistock Publications.

Calnan, M. and Johnson, B. (1985) 'Health, health risks and inequalities: an exploratory study of women's perceptions', *Sociology of Health and Illness* 7 (1): 55–75.

Chrisman, N.J., (1977) 'The health-seeking process: an approach to the natural history of illness', *Culture, Medicine and Psychiatry* 1 (4): 351–77.

Cornwell, J. (1984) *Hard-earned lives*, London: Tavistock Publications.

Crawford, R. (1977) 'You are dangerous to your health: the ideology and politics of victim-blaming', *International Journal of Health Services* 7 (4): 663–80.

Crawford, R. (1980) 'Healthism and the medicalization of everyday life', *International Journal of Health Services* 10 (3): 365–88.

Crawford, R. (1984) 'A cultural account of 'health': control, release, and the social body', in McKinley, J.B. (ed.) *Issues in the political economy of health care*, New York, London: Tavistock Publications, 60–103.

Desrosières, A. and Thévenot, L. (1988) *Les catégories socio-professionnelles*, Paris: Editions La Découverte.

D'Houtaud, A. and Field, M.G. (1984) 'The image of health: variations in perception by social class in a French population', *Sociology of Health and Illness* 6 (1): 30–60.

Dodier, N. (1984) *Une construction sociale précaire du biologique. Maladie et vie quotidienne sur le lieu de travail*, thèse pour le doctorat de sociologie, Paris: EHESS.

Fainzang, S. (1989) 'La santé: une affaire de médecins?', in D'Houtaud, A., Field, M. and Guéguen, R. (eds) *Les représentations de la santé. Bilan actuel, nouveaux développements*, Paris: INSERM 178: 435–9.

Fitzpatrick, R. (1984) 'Lay concepts of illness', in Fitzpatrick, R., Hinton, J., Newman, S., Scambler G. and Thompson, J. (eds) *The Experience of Illness*, London and New York: Tavistock Publications, 11–31.

Gallagher, E.B. (1976) 'Lines of reconstruction and extension in the Parsonian sociology of illness', *Social Science and Medicine* 10: 207–18.

Gerhardt, U. (1978) 'The Parsonian paradigm and the identity of medical sociology', *Sociological Review* 27 (2): 229–51.

Gerson, E.M. (1976) 'The social character of illness: deviance or politics?', *Social Science and Medicine* 10: 219–24.

Grossman, M. (1972) *The demand for health, a theoretical and empirical investigation*, New York: Columbia University Press.

Helman, C.G. (1978) ' "Feed a cold, starve a fever" folk models of infection in an English suburban community and their relation to medical treatment', *Culture, Medicine and Psychiatry* 2 (2): 107–37.

Herzlich, C. (1973) *Health and Illness*, London: Academic Press.

Herzlich, C. (1984a) 'Médecine moderne et quête de sens: la maladie signifiant social', in Augé, M. and Herzlich, C. (eds) *Le sens du mal. Anthropologie, histoire, sociologie de la maladie*, Paris: Editions des Archives Contemporaines, 189–215, English translation forthcoming, *The meaning of illness*, Reading: Gordon and Breach.

Herzlich, C. (1984b) 'La problématique de la représentation sociale et son utilité dans le champ de la maladie', *Sciences Sociales et Santé* 2 (2): 71–84.

Herzlich, C. and Pierret, J. (1987) *Illness and Self in Society*, Baltimore: Johns Hopkins University.

Hunt, S.M. and McEwen, J. (1980) 'The development of a subjective health indicator', *Sociology of Health and Illness* 2: 231–46.

Jodelet, D. (1989) 'Représentations sociales: un domaine en expansion' in Jodelet, D. (ed.) *Les représentations sociales*, Paris: PUF, 31–61.

Loux, F. and Richard, P. (1978) *Sagesse du corps: la santé et la maladie dans les proverbes français*, Paris: Maisonneuve-Larose.

Macintyre, S. (1986) 'The patterning of health by social position in contemporary Britain: directions for sociological research', *Social Science and Medicine* 23 (4): 393–415.

Moscovici, S. (1973) 'Foreword' in Herzlich, C. (1973) *Health and Illness*, London: Academic Press, ix-xiv.

Pierret, J. (1984) 'Les significations sociales de la santé: Paris, l'Essonne, l'Hérault' in Augé, M. and Herzlich, C. (eds) *Le sens du mal. Anthropologie, histoire, sociologie de la maladie*, Paris: Editions des Archives Contemporaines, 217–56, English translation forthcoming, *The meaning of illness*, Reading: Gordon and Breach.

Pierret, J. (1988) 'What social groups think they can do about health' in Anderson, R., Davies, J.K., Kickbusch, I., McQueen, D.V. and Turner, J. (eds) *Health Behaviour Research and Health Promotion*, Oxford University Press, 45–52.

Pill, R. and Stott, N.C.H. (1982) 'Concepts of illness causation and responsibility: some preliminary data from a sample of working class mothers', *Social Science and Medicine* 16 (1): 43–52.

Radley, A. (1988) *Prospects of Heart Surgery. Psychological Adjustment to Coronary Bypass Grafting*, New York: Springer-Verlag.

Radley, A. and Green, R. (1987) 'Illness as adjustment: a methodology and conceptual framework', *Sociology of Health and Illness* 9 (2): 179–207.

Renaud, M. (1981) 'Les réformes québécoises de la santé ou les aventures d'un État narcissique' in Bozzini, L., Renaud, M., Gaucher, D. and Llambias-Wolff, J. (eds) *Médecine et société. Les années 80*, Montréal: Editions Saint-Martin, 513–49.

Schneider, J.W. and Conrad, P. (1983) *Having Epilepsy: The Experience and Control of Illness*, Philadelphia: Temple University Press.

Speedling, E. (1982) *Heart Attack. The family response at home and in the hospital*, London and New York: Tavistock Publications.

Stacey, M. (1976) 'Concepts of health and illness. A working paper on the concepts and their relevance for research', University of Warwick, paper for 'Health and Health Policy', panel of the Social Science Research Council.

Stacey, M. (1986) 'Concepts of health and illness and the division of labour in health care' in Currer, C. and Stacey, M. (eds) *Concepts of health, illness and disease. A comparative perspective*, Leamington Spa, Hamburg and New York: Berg Publishers Ltd, 9–26.

Strauss, A.L. and Glaser, B.G. (eds) (1975) *Chronic Illness and the Quality of Life*, St Louis: Mosby.

Townsend, P. and Davidson, N. (1982) *Inequalities in health: the Black Report*, Harmondsworth: Penguin Books.

Williams, R.G.A. (1981) 'Logical analysis as a qualitative method I: themes in old age and chronic illness' and 'Logical analysis as a qualitative method II: conflict of ideas and the topic of illness', *Sociology of Health and Illness* 3 (2): 140–64 and 165–87.

Williams, R.G.A. (1983) 'Concepts of Health: an analysis of lay logic', *Sociology* 17: 185–204.

Williams, R.G.A. (1990) *A protestant legacy. Attitudes to death and illness among older Aberdonians*, Oxford: Clarendon Press.

Zola, I.K. (1977) 'Healthism and Disabling Medicalization' in Illich, I., Zola, I.K., McKnight, J., Caplan, J. and Shziken, H. (eds) *Disabling Professions*, London: Marion Boyars Publ. Ltd, 41–67.

2 Social class and the contextualization of illness experience

Alan Blair

INTRODUCTION

Overview

The object of this chapter is threefold. First, a theoretical rationale will be outlined which underpins the construction of a predictive model of social-class differences in the experience and communication of distress. Distress here is meant in the widest sense, referring to the set of all possible physical, cognitive and affective experiences. Second, a series of studies will be presented which attempt to address this model. Finally, the implications of these findings will be addressed, particularly within the context of the medical sociology literature.

Culture and distress

If the relationship between social class and the experience of distress is taken as the analytical problem, as it is in this chapter, there are a number of possible starting points for a social scientific inquiry.

One such starting point is to consider work within the fields of 'ethno-medicine' (e.g. Fabrega 1977) and the 'new cross-cultural psychiatry' (e.g. Kleinman 1977). While it seems that for a number of years the orthodoxy in medical and psychiatric theory and practice was one of cultural equivalence in the experience of distress, workers such as Kleinman and Fabrega have sought to emphasize the importance of culture in shaping differences in such experience.

Central to the theoretical formulations of these workers was a distinction between the form and content of distress. Indeed, Kiev (1972), for example, has made this point explicitly. While the form of psychiatric disorders was seen by Kiev as remaining essentially constant across cultures and time, the content of their expression is 'influenced' or 'shaped' by such culturally-specific features as the prevailing explanatory models of illness, the experience of self and the organization of the health-care system.

Although such work has proved an important and significant development, it may be that the form-content distinction is an unnecessary one. An ethnographic level of analysis, it can be contended, should always be orientated towards the location of forms of distress within specific linguistic frameworks and sets of historically-grounded cultural practices. From this standpoint, all forms of distress can be interpreted as 'culture-bound', and the essentialist position implicit in a form/content distinction is rendered fairly meaningless. The work of Mishler and colleagues (Mishler *et al.* 1981), Foucault (1967, 1973, 1976) and Wright and Treacher (1982), for example, has served to highlight the importance, for a full understanding of the experience of distress, of locating Western medical and psychiatric practices within their own social and historical contexts.

Related to the above, Szasz (1961) has contended that the very language of illness and disease has particular implications for the way in which distress is expressed and managed. Indeed, Waissman (1968) has argued for the central significance of language in determining experience. Language, rather than simply serving to report facts, was viewed as a 'collective instrument of thought that enters experience itself, shaping and moulding the whole apprehension of phenomena' (Waissman 1968: 175) (cf. Whorf 1956).

Following Waissman, Needham (1972) suggested a central role for language in the construction of selfhood, suggesting that the individual is subject to the influence of language in 'the most personal situation', namely the expression of their inner state of mind (Needham 1972: 238). Indeed, elsewhere Needham has called for 'a comprehensive knowledge of the values, collective representations, modes of organization and so on which comprise society' (Needham 1981: 67) in order to understand the construction of mind and has argued that the inner state must be viewed as a 'social fact' (Needham 1981: 71).

A number of authors have identified the differing conceptions of 'self' in their identification of cultural and historical differences in the experience of distress. Marsella (1984: 362), for example, contended that mental disorders cannot be understood apart from the concept of self, primarily because it was the nature of self which served in the identification of reality for a given cultural group and which dictated the definition of what was to be a symptom (cf. Shweder and Bourne, 1984). For example, within Western cultures, consciousness has been conceptualized as relatively more 'reflexive' (e.g. Dreitzel 1981: 221) and 'internalised' (e.g. Heelas 1981: 8) than non-Western cultures.

Thus, what such workers have chosen to emphasize is the importance of the relationship between language and the social construction of self in determining experience. However, what is also required is the explication of a general theoretical framework to articulate some of the dynamics of this relationship. To this end, it will be argued that the work of Volosinov (e.g. 1973, 1976), who has specifically addressed the relationship between language, ideology and consciousness, may prove of some utility.

The social construction of consciousness

Volosinov, whose work has been located in the context of the 'Baxtin Group' (Titunik 1973), made an explicit attempt to engage in what he argued was a central task of Marxism, namely the construction of 'a genuinely objective psychology' (Volosinov 1973: 25).

From the perspective of semiotics, Volosinov contended that individual consciousness only arises and becomes viable in 'the material embodiment of signs' through the process of social interaction, and that it requires to be understood as a 'socio-ideological fact' (Volosinov 1973: 11–12). Objective psychology for Volosinov had, therefore, to be grounded in the study of ideologies. Thus, he argued,

> Consciousness takes shape and being in the material of signs created by an organized group in the process of its social intercourse. The individual consciousness is nurtured on signs; it derives its growth from them; it reflects their logic and laws. The logic of consciousness is the logic of ideological communication, of the semiotic interaction of the social group. If we deprive consciousness of its semiotic, ideological content, it would have absolutely nothing left.
>
> (Volosinov, 1973: 13)

Locating consciousness within the domain of social interaction, as Volosinov did, has important ramifications for the understanding of individual experience. Production relations and the sociopolitical order shaped by those relations were conceptualized as the basis upon which the full range of verbal contacts, and thus individual consciousness, was determined. From this perspective, Volosinov contended that the processes that basically define the content of the psyche occur not inside but outside the individual organism and that a psychic phenomenon becomes explainable solely in terms of 'the social factors that shape the concrete life of the individual in the conditions of his social environment' (Volosinov 1973: 25–6).

Experience, for Volosinov, only existed in the material of signs and, thus, he contended that there was no qualitative difference between inner experience and the expression, or communication, of that experience (Volosinov 1973: 28) (cf. Marsella 1984: 363). The 'individual' was conceptualized as a socioideological phenomenon and, thus, individual consciousness was located within a set of social relations which are historically and culturally determined.

Taking such a stance, we can begin to address the analytical problem of social class and its relationship to consciousness generally and the experience of distress in particular. What is needed, however, are details of the contexts within and through which class-based experience emerges and the ways in which such contexts might specifically produce or constrain such experience. Of relevance here is the work of Basil Bernstein.

Social class and sociolinguistic codes

Influenced particularly by the work of Durkheim (e.g. 1915) and Sapir (e.g. 1929), Bernstein's 'special concern', in the words of Douglas (1973: 41), was to discover 'how speech forms transform the experience of speakers'. Bernstein argued that such speech forms were generated in social relations, which, by their selection and emphases, exercised a constraining effect on social behaviour.

From this theoretical background, Bernstein proposed two basic categories of sociolinguistic 'code', namely restricted and elaborated, and he identified a propensity towards the utilisation of these two codes in the working and middle class respectively. He posited that 'different speech systems or codes create for their speakers different orders of relevance and relation' and that experience is then 'transformed by what is made significant or relevant by the different speech systems' (Bernstein 1974: 174).

That Bernstein specifically chose social class to differentiate between levels of utilisation of the two codes was due to the primary significance he gave to class as a formative influence on the 'procedures of socialization'. The class structure, he argued, influenced both work and educational roles, bringing families into a 'special relationship with each other' and it deeply penetrated 'the structure of life experiences within the family' (cf. Kohn 1969). Moreover, the class system was viewed as significantly affecting the distribution of knowledge within society. It gave 'differential access to the sense that the world is permeable', it 'sealed off communities from each other', and it 'ranked these communities on a scale of invidious worth' (Bernstein 1974: 175). Indeed, it is in the arenas of power and control that the utilization of the elaborated code was viewed as predominating.

Given the above, it can be argued that Bernstein's sociolinguistic approach can be broadly located within Volosinov's theoretical conceptualization of the construction of consciousness. The experience of different social class groups within Britain today was, for Bernstein, a product of their differing positions within the set of social and economic relations. The articulation of a model of how this might specifically influence the experience of distress is the task of the next section.

CLASS, CODES AND DISTRESS

Bernstein has discussed some of the implications that the two codes might have for the behaviour and experience of the individual. An elaborated code was conceived of as becoming a facility for the transmission of 'individuated verbal responses'. The concept of self will, it was argued, becomes verbally differentiated in such a manner that it becomes in itself the object of 'special perceptual activity'. This can be seen as contrasting with the experience of a speaker relatively limited to a restricted code. In this case, the concept of self, through the implications of 'status arrangements', will tend to become 'refracted' (Bernstein 1974: 132).

Through the early orientation of the middle-class child towards the 'verbal channel', he comes to perceive of language as 'a set of theoretical possibilities for the presentation of his discrete experience to others'. The elaborated code thus induces, developmentally, an 'expectation of separateness and difference from others' in its speakers (Bernstein 1974: 133).

We can see the significance of such a conceptualization by opposing it to a description of the experience of speakers more oriented towards using the restricted code. Speech for such users was not generally conceived of as becoming the object of special perceptual activity. This, for Bernstein, had critical implications if the reference was to the subjective state of the speaker. He contended that, although such speech possessed a warmth and intensity, it tended to be impersonal in the literal sense of the word. The original social relation between parent and child was viewed as exerting little pressure on the child to make her experience relatively explicit in a verbally differentiated way. Most importantly:

> Speech is not perceived as a major means of presenting to the other inner states. The type of learning, the conditions of learning and the dimensions of relevance initiated and sustained through a restricted code are radically different from the learning induced through an elaborated code.
>
> (Bernstein 1974: 134)

If, as Bernstein has argued, subjective experience, the concept of self, and the articulation and elaboration of 'inner states' differs between the users of the two codes, then a fairly direct link can be made to an hypothesis about class differences in the experience and communication of distress. Working class 'tensions', for Bernstein, were more likely to be articulated through more immediate, proximal channels of expression, such as 'changes in muscular tension, somato–motor set, or expressive behaviour' (1964: 61).

Thus, it is suggested that, for the working class, distress will typically be experienced and communicated in a relatively proximal, localized immediate way – that is, through the medium of the body. For the middle class, contrastingly, it is suggested that distress is more likely to be experienced in individuated, personalized ways. There is more emphasis on a unique mental life which can be differentiated from others. Thus, for the middle class, distress will be relatively more psychically (as opposed to physically) mediated (see Table 2.1).

Table 2.1 Hypothesized relationship between social class and the predominant site of distress

Class	*Code*	*Experience of self*	*Site of distress*
Working class	Restricted	Positional Proximal	Body
Middle class	Elaborated	Personal Differentiated	Psyche

Of course, the work of Bernstein has not been without its critics (e.g. Labov 1970; Rosen 1973; Robinson 1979), criticisms which have been considered elsewhere (Atkinson 1985; Blair 1986). However, what is of concern here is the articulation of a general theoretical position and the development of a predictive model. In this sense, Bernstein's approach can be used as a heuristic device for theorizing about class differences in the experience and communication of distress.

On the basis of the general hypothesis that the working class are relatively more preoccupied with the body as a site of distress experience and that middle-class respondents are relatively more preoccupied with the psyche as a site of such experience, four studies were undertaken which are summarized below and reported in full in Blair (1986). All studies were conducted by a male Caucasian researcher in East Sussex, England, during 1985 or 1986.

STUDIES OF THE RELATIONSHIP BETWEEN SOCIAL CLASS AND THE EXPERIENCE OF DISTRESS

Reported experience

In Study 1, 118 respondents were approached either in their workplace or at home. Respondents were told that the interview was on the subject of 'how they had been feeling over the last week or so'. Specifically, respondents were asked questions on how they had been feeling for each of the last four days as well as a fifth question on how they had been feeling in general over the last week. Those whose answers were very short, particularly single word replies (e.g. 'alright'), were given an additional prompting question by the interviewer in order to encourage further talk. Interviews lasted a mean of approximately four minutes (ranging from two to twenty minutes).

Using occupational information gained within the interview, respondents were classified in this and subsequent studies as belonging to one of two social-class categories, namely working class or middle class. Occupation was initially coded utilizing Erikson, Goldthorpe and Portocarero's (1979) extended eleven-fold schema. This schema was subsequently collapsed into two social-class categories, following the rationale of Goldthorpe (1980), particularly his conceptualization of the 'service class' drawn from Renner (1953) and his distinction between salaried and waged. A full description of this procedure is given elsewhere (Blair 1986).

Each interview script was analysed for the occurrence of 'experience terms'. An experience term was recorded for each occasion that a respondent used a word or phrase which, within the context of the dialogue, appeared to describe a feeling, mood, state, bodily sensation, bodily disorder and/or category of illness.

Each experience term was then designated as belonging to one of three discrete categories, namely predominantly physically located experience (a 'physicalistic' term), predominantly mentally located experience (a 'mentalistic' term) or ambiguous. Experience terms were coded as physicalistic when they appeared to refer to bodily sensations and disorders or to categories of physical illness experience (e.g. pains, aches, physical tiredness, influenza, etc.). Contrastingly, experience terms were coded as mentalistic when they appeared to refer to psychic and/or emotional experience (e.g. happy, scared, depressed, under pressure, etc.). There was a high level of cross-coder reliability in the coding of terms.

Broadly consistent with hypotheses, it was found that working-class respondents used slightly but significantly more physicalistic terms than middle-class respondents. On average, working-class respondents used approximately three such terms while middle-class respondents used approximately two. Contrastingly, middle-class respondents used considerably and significantly more mentalistic terms (approximately 6.5) than working-class respondents (approximately 2).

Additional analyses included the construction of sub-categories. While significant class differences were found in each of the four mentalistic sub-categories, class differences were particularly marked in the sub-categories of 'negative elaborated mentalistic experience' and 'positive elaborated mentalistic experience'. Examples of experience terms in the former sub-category included 'everything's falling in upon my head', 'feel in need of a break', and 'feel I was wasting my time'. While 29 per cent of middle-class respondents used at least one term in this category, only 5 per cent of working-class respondents did so. Examples of experience terms in the latter sub-category included 'feel a sense of modified well-being', 'feel at peace with myself' and 'feel how nice it was to be on my own'. While 38 per cent of middle-class respondents used at least one term in this category, only 10 per cent of working-class respondents did so.

Additionally to the above, it was found that middle-class respondents used two specific mentalistic terms to a significantly greater extent, namely 'depressed' and 'worried'. There was no significant class difference between use of terms coded as ambiguous.

Given the above, it was concluded that there were marked and predictable social-class differences in people's talk in response to questions about how they had been feeling. Indeed, given that middle-class respondents used more experience terms overall, it appeared that the research situation was one in which the middle class were willing to engage in more verbal activity: i.e. that the research was conducted within contexts in which middle-class respondents had more to speak about or felt greater ease in speaking.

Specifically, it is contended that the reason that middle-class respondents typically talked at greater length in response to questions about how they had been feeling recently is related to the sociolinguistic codes with which they typically operate. The middle class, it is suggested, are more oriented towards individualized, differentiated experience and thus concern themselves more with personalized feelings, sentiments, moods and so on. They are likely to engage in more self-reflective activity, and will be more oriented towards dialogues in which their own feelings are a topic of discussion.

To give a flavour of the differences between social classes, four representative scripts are reprinted in full. The first two are of interviews with middle-class respondents (Dave and Ann), the next two are of interviews with working-class respondents (Pam and Ian). The names of respondents are fictitious.

1. Middle-class male (Dave)

Int.: How are you feeling today?

Dave: Eh, a bit sort of panicky.

Int.: Can you say any more about how you are feeling today?

Dave: Em, quite happy, a bit excited, and I was feeling a bit depressed earlier on.

Int.: Do you remember how you were feeling yesterday, on Sunday?

Dave: I was feeling a bit down in the morning, but then I was feeling happy for the rest of the day.

Int.: Do you remember how you were feeling on Saturday, at the beginning of the weekend?

Dave: Em, I was generally feeling in a good mood. Happy, but then I felt a bit down in the afternoon, and very tired in the evening.

Int.: Do you remember how you were feeling last Friday?

Dave: Last Friday, em I can't remember what I was doing last Friday. Ah yes, I was feeling a bit depressed for most of the day, but then I felt really happy in the evening.

Int.: Over the last week or so how have you been feeling in general?

Dave: Up and down.

Int.: Can you say any more about how you've been feeling over the last week or so?

Dave: Em, not really. It's fluctuated between feeling a bit depressed and feeling very happy. Feeling, em, a bit panicky because of work, feeling tired sometimes, and other times feeling full of energy. That's about it.

2. Middle-class female (Ann)

Int.: How are you feeling today?

Ann: Dreadful. Yes, depressed, tired, busy. I'm suffering from post-operational depression. Had an operation nearly a month ago and still feel really down. I get odd bright half hours, you know, but I don't feel good. Very, very down indeed. Em, generally very lethargic, very tired. Spending three-quarters of my life sleeping at the moment. Em, not very happy about anything at all.

Int.: Do you remember how you were feeling yesterday, on Monday?

Ann: Marginally better yesterday. Em, I felt quite cheerful for about two hours. Then it hit me again. No haven't really felt good for a month, not since I had the operation. It was only a tiny one, but it has really shaken my body up.

Int.: How were you feeling on Sunday?

Ann: Dreadful. Em, incredibly tired. Spent most of the day in bed sleeping, feeling very sorry for myself. Em, very low, very unhappy.

Int.: How were you feeling on Saturday?

Ann: Yes, weepy. I had to do the shopping and I felt really, I really wanted to weep. I didn't want to do it. Em, very bad indeed, Saturday was a very bad day. But Monday was quite good.

Int.: Over the last week or so in general how have you been feeling?

Ann: Up and down. Em, generally low, generally not terribly happy about life. Sort of feeling I ought to be doing things and not being able to do them. Not very pleased about my lack of enthusiasm, either at work or anything at home, or anything at all for that matter.

3. Working-class female (Pam)

Int.: How are you feeling today?

Pam: Alright, apart from a sore throat, cos I discovered the past couple of weeks that I've got an allergy, you see. I'm allergic to something. So I've got to find out what it is.

Int.: Can you say any more about how you are feeling today?

Pam: Alright, the same as usual.

Int.: Do you remember how you were feeling yesterday, on Sunday?

Pam: Same as today.

Int.: Which is?

Pam: Usual.

Int.: How you were feeling on Saturday?

Pam: Saturday? No different as what, to what I am now really, you know.

Int.: So, how were you feeling on Saturday?

Pam: I don't know what you want me to answer, 'cos I mean I haven't been any different as what I've been, what a week or two weeks, apart from, you know, this allergy I've got, whatever it is.

Int.: Do you want to say anything about how you were feeling on Friday?

Pam: Worn out.

Int.: In general over the last week or so how have you been feeling?

Pam: Alright. Myself really, apart from, you know, feeling slightly sick. That's been getting me down a little bit. But, apart from that, alright.

4. Working-class male (Ian)

Int.: How are you feeling today?

Ian: Feeling alright.

Int.: Can you say any more about how you are feeling today?

Ian: No. I just feel happy, and I've got me kids and I've got me work. I feel alright.

Int.: Do you remember how you were feeling yesterday, on Sunday?

Ian: Yeah, I felt alright.

Int.: Again, can you say any more about how you were feeling on Sunday?

Ian: Not really, no. Just feel the same.

Int.: Can you say anything about how you were feeling on Friday?

Ian: No

Int.: So, in general over the last week or so how have you been feeling?

Ian: No different really.
Int.: How was that you were feeling?
Ian: No different from what I usually feel.
Int.: Which is what?
Ian: Quite normal.

Of course, there are a number of possible interpretations and qualifications of the above data other than those forwarded. These have been considered elsewhere (Blair 1986) and include interviewer effects, lack of generalizability to other questions and lack of generalizability to other contexts. In addition, it could be argued that the observed class differences could be accounted for by either or both middle-class respondents finding it relatively more socially acceptable to express emotional difficulties in the research context and/or working-class respondents living and working in conditions which are likely to cause more physical illness and injury. An attempt to partially counter such alternative accounts was made in Study 2.

THEORIES OF DISTRESS

Of central interest in Study 2 were class differences in individuals' theories about the nature of, aetiology of and methods of coping with distress. This was done through depersonalizing the content of questioning in ways which, it was anticipated, would reduce the likelihood of any observed differences being a consequence of the effects of social desirability or individuals' material conditions.

In this study ninety-eight respondents were interviewed either in their workplace or at home. Respondents were read one of two vignettes which consisted of a description of an individual with a collection of symptoms which were open to theorizing about in either physicalistic or mentalistic terms. In both vignettes allusions were made to possible psychological causes of a person's distress. Both vignettes are reprinted in full below.

Vignette 1

Let's suppose you have a neighbour who is a middle-aged father of three. He works in a busy office. Recently he has begun to complain a lot of headaches and dizziness and he has been finding that often his heart seems to beat very quickly and irregularly. When you last spoke to him he told you that he seems to get tired much easier than he used to and often he finds trouble in getting to sleep at night. He says he finds it difficult to keep up with things at work at the moment and he also seems quite worried about his ill-health.

Vignette 2

Let's suppose you have a neighbour who is a thirty-year-old married mother of four, who works nights part-time in a hospital. For the last few years she has suffered from blinding headaches off and on and these seem to have become more frequent recently. Often when she gets these headaches she is sick and gets diarrhoea. When she feels this way she finds it difficult to do any work and she will often have to lie down for a few hours until it wears off.

Following presentation of these vignettes, respondents were asked a series of questions tapping various aspects of their theories about such experiences, their answers being subsequently analysed in terms of social-class differences. It was found that while 75 per cent of working-class respondents gave relatively physicalistic accounts of the aetiology of the distress described in the presented vignette, 76 per cent of middle-class respondents gave relatively mentalistic accounts. Particularly common among working-class respondents were accounts in terms of 'circulatory disorders' and 'tiredness'. Contrastingly, particularly common among middle-class respondents were accounts in terms of 'stress' and 'anxiety'.

Not surprisingly, given the above, there were class differences in the strategies which respondents felt would have been useful for avoiding the presented distress. Middle-class respondents, for example, were significantly more likely to suggest that 'the expression of feelings' would have been helpful, while working-class respondents were more likely to suggest 'taking things easier'.

Turning to treatments of the distress described in the vignettes, it was found that, while over one-third of working-class respondents gave considerable efficacy to physicalistic treatments, only 2 per cent of middle-class respondents did so. Contrastingly, 68 per cent of middle-class respondents gave considerable efficacy to mentalistic treatments, while only 8 per cent of working-class respondents did so. More specifically, middle-class respondents were significantly more likely to make positive mention of 'therapy and talking' and 'personal change', while working-class respondents were significantly more likely to make positive mention of 'medical treatments'.

Such results suggested that there were powerful class differences in the way in which ambiguous experiences of distress are interpreted, in the theories which are forwarded to account for such distress and in the remedies suggested for the alleviation of such distress. However, two qualifications need to be made. First, it was not clear the extent to which these class differences would generalize to distress of a less ambiguous nature. Second it was not clear the extent to which the very act of labelling the distress presented in the vignettes shaped both the theories of causality and also the proposed remedies. Thus, two further studies were carried out which, rather than presenting ambiguous vignettes, held the distress label constant: in Study 3, the relatively physicalistic experience of cancer and in Study 4, the relatively mentalistic experience of depression.

Representations of cancer

Cancer, which is frequently used as a general disease category (Sontag 1979), is an increasingly prevalent group of diseases in Western industrial societies (e.g. American Cancer Society 1978) and individuals' attitudes towards and beliefs about cancer have become the object of much research (e.g. Wortman and Dunkel-Schetter 1979; Linn *et al.* 1982). However, relatively few have considered whether any class differences exist in such representations of cancer.

In this study fifty respondents were interviewed either in their workplace or at an adult education class (upholstery, keep fit or woodwork). Respondents were given a standard set of twelve questions, either open-ended or asking for a score of between 1 and 10, on their 'opinions about cancer'. Interviews lasted a mean of twelve minutes.

Looking at representations of the aetiology of cancer, it was found that middle-class respondents used a variety of relatively mentalistic accounts to a significantly greater extent than working-class respondents, including 'stress', 'anxiety or worry', being in 'poor psychological condition' and 'not expressing feelings'. Contrastingly, the accounts used to a significantly greater extent by working-class respondents were relatively physicalistic in orientation, namely 'dust', 'pollution', 'too much alcohol', 'smoking', being 'overweight' and 'poisonous chemicals'.

Turning to respondents' perceptions of the efficacy of physicalistic and mentalistic treatments, it was found that, while, on average, working-class respondents gave slightly higher ratings of the efficacy of physicalistic treatments, the difference was not significant. However, there was a large and significant class difference in the perceived efficacy of mentalistic treatments, with, on average, middle class respondents scoring the efficacy of such treatments 7 (out of 10) and working-class respondents scoring such efficacy only 2.4.

More particularly, middle-class respondents made more frequent positive mention of 'therapy and talking', 'fighting it psychologically', 'having support from family and friends', 'belief in treatment', 'adopting a positive attitude' and 'seeking information about cancer'. Indeed, important for many middle-class individuals was the role of self in combating the progress of cancer. Typical of such responses were the following excerpts from scripts:

> 'I think willpower is the most important factor because ... there's no real cure .... The only thing they need to do is to realize what they've got and try and combat it ... by willpower rather than by anything else, but if you give in, you give in. If you fight then you stand a chance to win.'

> 'There must be probably a psychological side .... It probably depends upon the actual person's mentality. You probably have to be a strong sort of person to help yourself in that situation ... a great factor is your own willpower in overcoming it ... not just cancer, I mean in anything you have, in any disability, it is your own personality basically that some people recover more and get back more punch than others. They put more into their recovery don't they? ... It's down to you really.'

By contrast, working-class respondents gave less value to personal control and, indeed, made significantly more positive mention of such physically-based treatments as 'surgery' and 'drugs'. In addition, working-class respondents were significantly more likely to answer that 'no help or advice' was possible and that any recovery was a matter of 'luck'. Typical of such responses were the following two excerpts from scripts:

> 'I don't rightly think you have any control really. Once you've got it you've got it, and the medical side it may help but there again it's as likely not to help, so I don't see how you've got any control. You've just got to cross your fingers and hope for the best.'

> 'Once cancer gets a grip you've just to go to wait and hope, take the drugs and the treatment and what have you, rest a lot, and hope that it goes away, but there's not a lot of control you have over it.'

Not surprisingly, given the above, there were significant class differences in respondents' estimates of individuals' control over the course of cancer. Middle-class respondents gave a mean score of 5.6 (out of 10) compared with working-class respondents' mean score of 3.3.

Representations of depression

In order to assess the generalizability of such results to other types of distress, a final study addressed individuals' representations of depression. In this study 79 respondents completed a questionnaire while attending a community school 'Open Day'. Similarly to Study 3, respondents were asked a standard set of twelve questions, about their 'opinions about depression'.

Looking at representations of the aetiology of depression, it was again found that middle-class respondents used a variety of relatively mentalistic accounts to a significantly greater extent than working-class respondents, such accounts being of two major types. First, there were accounts for which responsibility could be located largely within the individual, including 'unrealistic expectations', 'bottling up feelings', 'lack of self-esteem' and 'too self-critical' and, second, there were accounts which located responsibility relatively more upon environmental pressures, including 'lack of a close relationship', 'death of someone close', 'unemployment' and 'major happenings in life'. Contrastingly, the accounts used to a significantly greater extent by working-class respondents were generally more physicalistic in orientation, including 'brain defect', 'hereditary', 'tiredness' and 'allergies'.

Turning to respondents' perceptions of the efficacy of physicalistic and mentalistic treatments, it was found that, working-class respondents gave significantly higher ratings to the efficacy of physicalistic treatments. On the other hand, middle-class respondents gave significantly higher ratings to the efficacy of mentalistic treatments.

More particularly, significantly more working-class respondents reported feeling that 'drugs', 'hospitalization', 'surgery', 'e. c. t.' and 'letting it take its own course' were useful strategies to deal with depression. Contrastingly, significantly more middle-class respondents reported feeling that individually facilitated change, such as 'adopting different attitude', 'meditation' and 'new hobbies and interests', or interaction with others, such as 'counselling', 'talking to local pastor' and 'talking to friend/relative', were useful strategies to deal with depression.

As in Study 3, there were significant class differences in respondent's estimates of individuals' control over the course of depression. Middle-class respondents gave a mean score of 6.4 (out of 10) compared with working class respondents' mean score of 4.5. For example, the following is typical of middle class responses:

> 'If they can be persuaded to concentrate their minds on the problem the solution has to ultimately come from within.'

> 'I feel people ultimately are the ones who have to cure themselves with an effort of will.'

By comparison, working-class respondents saw less role for individual control. For example:

> 'It's in the hands of the doctors and drugs really.'

Discussion

> 'I woke up one morning and I couldn't breathe. So, of course, I figured it

> was psycho-somatic. A free flowing withdrawal from unhappy visions. After that I developed a heaviness in my chest. So, of course, I figured it was psycho-somatic. A masochistic act of self-reproval towards my body. Then I got this gosh awful sneeze. So, of course, I figured it was psycho-somatic. An acting out, through germs, of my latent hostility towards society. Naturally, I grew worried about my emotional well-being. I went to see a psychiatrist. He told me I had a cold.
>
> (Feiffer 1960; cited in Bart 1968: 188)

The above quote was originally used by Bart (1968) to describe the increasing preoccupation of the 'educated circles' with the psyche as the site of distress. For Bart, as in this chapter, this was seen as having ramifications both for representations of distress aetiology and also for the choices individuals made about coping strategies and treatment.

Throughout this chapter, an attempt has been made to argue that an understanding of consciousness and, more specifically, the experience and communication of distress requires a theoretical model which emphasizes the contextual nature of such experience. From the above studies, it appears that Bernstein's (e.g. 1974) distinction between the restricted and elaborated code has provided a useful heuristic for predicting social-class differences in how such distress is expressed. Not only do middle-class respondents, relative to working-class respondents, appear to use more mentalistic language in describing their personal experience of distress, but they also appear to interpret others' distress in more mentalistic terms, attribute more psychological causality to the onset of distress and give more value to psychological strategies for dealing with distress. Not surprisingly, such class differences resulted in the middle class perceiving relatively more personal control over the course of distress.

Such findings may have implications for a variety of fields of social scientific inquiry. One such field is that of social representations (e.g. Moscovici 1981) which views individuals' explanations as rooted in their 'shared social beliefs' (Moscovici and Hewstone 1983: 100). This broad perspective has provided a framework for a number of workers, most importantly Herzlich (e.g. 1973), to consider representations of various aspects of distress. What has seldom been considered in such work is the issue of social class, however, although D'Houtaud and Field (1984) found that non-manual classes conceived of health in more personalized, positive and expressive terms, while manual classes conceived of health in more negative, socialized and institutional terms. That such class differences exist suggests the need for incorporating more explicitly into social representational work the role of social class as an important determinant in the construction of such representations.

The findings presented in this present chapter can also be located within the more general framework of the medical sociology literature. For example, there is some evidence that psychosomatic disorders are experienced more frequently by the working class (e.g. Hollingshead and Redlich 1958). Indeed, Fried (1975) concluded that among the few findings which have emerged with any consistency in the literature on the relationship between social class and mental health is 'the emphasis on physical symptoms, physical interpretations of psychological symptoms, and an organic conception of psychiatric disorder among lower-class patients' (Fried 1975: 179). Similarly, Kleinman (1980) has detailed class differences in rates of 'somatization' which, he argued, are more prevalent among 'lower' class groups. Contrastingly. Kleinman contended that the American middle class are preoccupied with the 'psychologization' of distress.

Of course, the relationship between social class and rates of diagnosable mental and physical illness is complex and goes beyond the remit of this chapter. Nevertheless, what appears to be indicated is a need to consider such rates in the context of the typical ways in which individuals experience and communicate distress. Distress is inevitably socially constructed and mediated, not least through social class.

Such a contention also has implications for class differences in the take-up, allocation and efficacy of treatments for distress. For example, it has long been observed that the working class tend to present themselves relatively less frequently to psychological and psychiatric services (e.g. Hollingshead and Redlich 1958; Fink *et al.* 1970; Weissman and Myers 1978). A number of accounts have been forwarded to explain this, including Bart's (1968) proposition that the middle class have more access to 'psychiatric vocabularies of discomfort'.

Interestingly, social-class differences have also been found in the use of preventive services (e.g. Brotherston 1976; Calnan 1985), in which the role of personal agency and personal responsibility is an important determinant. As Pill and Stott (1982) have contended, what needs to be established are the social differences in the meaning of individual responsibility. For example, approximately half of their sample of working-class mothers were found to hold fatalistic views of the aetiology of illness. Indeed, similar observations have been made by workers using the health belief model (e.g. Rosenstock 1974). As Blaxter (1976: 123) has argued, 'There are many groups in the population whose position in the social structure makes it difficult for them to subscribe to that belief in the rational mastery of the world which typifies the professional approach' (cf. Gray 1979).

We can also see the effect of such social class differences in the allocation of mental health services, with psychotherapy appearing to be less frequently offered to working-class clients (e.g. Kandel 1966). Of course, the value system of the treatment allocator may have an impact upon allocation (e.g. McMahon 1964). Rowden *et al.* (1970), for example, found that 'high' social class and high 'insight-verbal' ability enhanced the probability of selection for psychotherapy, while Foon (1985) noted the importance of 'control orientation' in mediating between social class and therapists' expectations.

There is also some evidence, however, that because of the more physicalistic and less agentive orientation of working-class clients, psychotherapy, or at least some forms of psychotherapy, may be less effective. Returning to Basil Bernstein, he has argued that

> sensitivity to the psychotherapeutic relationship and the forms of communication considered to be appropriate is less available to members of the lower working class, not by virtue of innate deficiencies in intelligence but because of a culturally induced speech system whose dimensions of relevance and significance do not orient the working-class patient in the therapy relationship.
>
> (Bernstein, 1964: 194)

Bernstein conceived of the psychotherapeutic relationship as a form of social relationship in which 'tension' is exerted upon the patient 'to structure and restructure his discrete experience in a verbally significant form'. Thus,

> The referent for this communication is the patient – or rather his motivational processes and the implicit or explicit social relationships which they engender. The 'I' of the patient is undergoing a continuous transformation by virtue of those unique communications.
>
> (Bernstein, 1964: 195)

Moreover, for Bernstein, to the extent that the patient's communications are 'filtered' through the purposes, goals and beliefs of their 'natural group', the patient's appropriate self-perception is considered to be hindered. The conventions which, for Bernstein, were seen as conferring upon the working-class individual their social identity were viewed within the context of the psychotherapeutic relationship as material to be worked through in order to differentiate the individual from the group. Thus, Bernstein argued that successful therapy from this relatively middle-class standpoint was typically viewed as being based upon, '... mutual belief on the part of both therapist and patient that the illness may be removed by participation in a social relationship where the major activity is the transformation of discrete experience through the medium of communication, essentially through speech' (Bernstein 1964: 195).

Given the relative unusualness of this form of social relationship for the working class, Bernstein contended that such individuals will experience less benefit from therapy and will break off treatment earlier. Rather than being evidence of pathology or ignorance, he argued that this was entirely consistent with an orientation towards a different speech system, the restricted code. This, in sustaining social solidarity within the group, worked against the verbal elaboration of an individual's unique experience and relatively rarely considered the self as subject of elaborated verbal investigation. Such a position was also echoed by Shands and Meltzer (1973) and Meltzer (1978), the latter arguing that an understanding of the practice of psychotherapy required its location within contexts which emphasize the semiotic nature of such an enterprise (cf. Lacan 1968; Schafer 1976).

Given the above, it can be argued that psychotherapy has been developed within a largely middle-class frame of reference which is oriented towards a view of the individual which reflects the middle-class preoccupation with a differentiated psyche as the site of distress. Such an orientation appears from the literature to be relatively problematic when working with working-class clients. As Gallagher (1980), among others, has argued, there may be a need to re–examine psychotherapeutic techniques in ways which more fully take account of working-class experience. As summarized elsewhere (Blair 1986), among the alternatives forwarded are those which emphasize the role of the group rather than the individual, the social as opposed to the intrapsychic aetiology of distress and the role of action rather than introspection. Also in this context, recent advances in therapies which rely less on the need for extended verbal introspection for personal change, such as Neuro-Linguistic Programming (e.g. Bandler and Grinder 1979), may prove relevant.

To conclude, therefore, what has been attempted is an exposition and examination of a model of distress experience, which takes as a central tenet that consciousness is a socioideological construction. Returning to the opening sections of this chapter, it can be argued that distress cannot be understood without reference to the contexts of its experience and expression.

Too often, ill health, whether predominantly physical or mental, is decontextualized. The implicit assumption is that all individuals have an experience of distress which is essentially identical to that of white middle-class Western males. Within this chapter, however, the work of Basil Bernstein has been used to develop a model of the systematic way in which distress experience differs as a function of social class.

Of course, other cultural contexts not examined here, such as race and gender, are of equal if not greater significance. The general point, however, is to assert that distress experience requires to be firmly culturally located. To omit such a level of analysis from a consideration of any individual or group's experience is to fundamentally misrepresent the nature of such experience.

REFERENCES

American Cancer Society (1978) *1978 Facts and Figures*, New York: American Cancer Society.

Atkinson, P. (1985) *Language, Structure and Reproduction: An Introduction to the Sociology of Basil Bernstein*, London: Methuen.

Bandler, R. and Grinder, J. (1979) *Frogs Into Princes: Neuro Linguistic Programming*, Moab, Utah: Real People Press.

Bart, P. (1968) 'Social structure and vocabularies of discomfort: whatever happened to female hysteria?', *Journal of Health and Social Behavior* 9: 188–93.

Bernstein, B. (1964) 'Social class, speech systems, and psycho-therapy', *British Journal of Sociology* 15: 54–64.

Bernstein, B. (1974) *Class, Codes and Control. Volume 1: Theoretical Studies Towards a Sociology of Language*, London: Routledge & Kegan Paul.

Blair, A.J. (1986) 'Locating distress: social class and the contextualisation of illness experience', unpublished D. Phil. thesis, University of Sussex.

Blaxter, M. (1976) 'Social class and health inequalities', in C.O. Carter and J. Peel (eds) *Equalities and Inequalities in Health*, London: Academic Press.

Brotherston, J. (1976) 'Inequality: is it inevitable?', in C.O. Carter and J. Peel (eds) *Equalities and Inequalities in Health*, London: Academic Press.

Calnan, M. (1985) 'Patterns in preventative behaviour: a study of women in middle age', *Social Science and Medicine* 20: 263–8.

D'Houtaud, A. and Field, M.G. (1984) 'The image of health: variations in perceptions by social class in a French population', *Sociology of Health and Illness* 6: 30–60.

Douglas, M. (1973) *Natural Symbols: Explorations in Cosmology*, Harmondsworth: Penguin.

Dreitzel, H. (1981) 'The socialization of nature: Western attitudes towards the body and emotions', in P. Heelas and A. Lock (eds) *Indigenous Psychologies: The Anthropology of the Self*, London: Academic Press.

Durkheim, E. (1915) *Elementary Forms of the Religious Life*, London: Allen and Unwin.

Durkheim, E. (1933) *The Division of Labour in Society*, New York: Macmillan.

Erikson, R., Goldthorpe, J.H. and Portocarero, L. (1979) 'Intergenerational class mobility in three Western European societies: England, France and Sweden', *British Journal of Sociology* 30: 415–41.

Fabrega, H. (1977) 'The scope of ethnomedical science', *Culture, Medicine and Psychiatry* 1: 201–28.

Fink, R., Shapiro, S. and Goldensohn, S. (1970) 'Family physician referrals for psychiatric consultation and patient initiative in seeking care', *Social Science and Medicine* 4: 273–91.

Foon, A.E. (1985) 'The effect of social class and cognitive orientation on clinical expectations', *British Journal of Medical Psychology* 58: 357–64.

Foucault, M. (1967) *Madness and Civilization: A History of Insanity in the Age of Reason*, London: Tavistock Publications.

Foucault, M. (1973) *The Birth of the Clinic: An Archaeology of Medical Perception*, London: Tavistock Publications.

Foucault, M. (1976) *Mental Illness and Psychology*, New York: Harper & Row.

Fried, M. (1975) 'Social differences in mental health', in J. Kosa and I.K. Zola (eds) *Poverty and Health: A Sociological Analysis*, Cambridge, Ma.: Harvard University Press.

Gallagher, B.J. (1980) *The Sociology of Mental Illness*, Englewood-Cliffs, NJ: Prentice-Hall.

Goldthorpe, J.H. (1980) *Social Mobility and Class Structure in Modern Britain*, Oxford: Clarendon Press.

Gray, J.A.M. (1979) *Man Against Disease*, Oxford: Oxford University Press.

Heelas, P. (1981) 'Introduction: indigenous psychologies', in P. Heelas and A. Lock (eds) *Indigenous Psychologies: The Anthropology of the Self*, London: Academic Press.

Herzlich, C. (1973) *Health and Illness: A Social Psychological Analysis*, London: Academic Press.

Hollingshead, A.B. and Redlich, F.C. (1958) *Social Class and Mental Illness: A Community Study*, New York: Wiley.

Kandel, D.B. (1966) 'Status homiphily, social context, and participation in psychotherapy', *American Journal of Sociology* 71: 640–50.

Kiev, A. (1972) *Transcultural Psychiatry*, Glencoe: Free Press.

Kleinman, A. (1977) 'Depression, somatization, and the "new cross-cultural psychiatry" ', *Social Science and Medicine* 11: 85–93.

Kleinman, A. (1980) *Patients and Healers in the Context of Culture: An Exploration of the Borderland Between Anthropology, Medicine and Psychiatry*, Berkeley: University of California Press.

Kohn, M.L. (1969) *Class and Conformity*: A Study in Values, Homewood, Ill.: Dorsey Press.

Labov, W. (1970) 'The logic of non-standard English', in F. Williams (ed.) *Language and Poverty*, London: Markham Press.

Lacan, J. (1968) *The Language of Self: The Function of Language in Psychoanalysis*, Baltimore: Johns Hopkins University Press.

Linn, M.W., Linn, B.S. and Stein, S.R. (1982) 'Beliefs about causes of cancer in cancer patients', *Social Science and Medicine* 16: 835–9.

McMahon, J.T. (1964) 'The working class psychiatric patient: a clinical view', in F. Riessman, J. Cohen and A. Pearl (eds) *Mental Health of the Poor*, Glencoe: Free Press.

Marsella, A.J. (1984) 'Culture and mental health: an overview', in A.J. Marsella and G.M. White (eds) *Cultural Conceptions of Mental Health and Therapy*, Dordrecht: Reidel.

Meltzer, J.D. (1978) 'A semiotic approach to suitability for psychotherapy', *Psychiatry* 41: 360–76.

Mishler, E.G., Amarasingham, L.R., Osherson, S.D., Hauser, S.T., Waxler, N.E. and Liem, R. (1981) *Social Contexts of Health, Illness and Patient Care*, Cambridge: Cambridge University Press.

Moscovici, S. (1981) 'On social representations', in J.P. Forgas (ed.) *Social Cognition: Perspectives on Everyday Understanding*, London: Academic Press.

Moscovici, S. and Hewstone, M. (1983) 'Social representations and social explanations: from "naive" to "amateur" scientist', in M. Hewstone (ed.) *Attribution Theory: Social and Functional Extensions*, Oxford: Blackwell.

Needham, R. (1972) *Belief, Language and Experience*, Oxford: Blackwell.

Needham, R. (1981) 'Inner states as universals: sceptical reflections on human nature', in P. Heelas and A. Lock (eds) *Indigenous Psychologies: The Anthropology of the Self*, London: Academic Press.

Pill, R. and Stott, N.C.H. (1982) 'Concepts of illness causation and responsibility:

some preliminary data from a sample of working class mothers', *Social Science and Medicine* 16: 43–52.

Renner, K. (1953) *Wandlungen der Modernen Gesellschaft: Zwei abhandlungen uber die probleme der Nachkriegszeit*, Vienna.

Robinson, W.P. (1979) 'Speech markers and social class', in K.R. Scherer and H. Giles (eds) *Social Markers in Speech*, Cambridge: Cambridge University Press.

Rosen, H. (1973) *Language and Class: A Critical Look at the Theories of Basil Bernstein*, Bristol: Falling Wall Press.

Rosenstock, I.M. (1974) 'The health belief model and preventative behavior', *Health Education Monographs* 2: 354–86.

Rowden, D.W., Michel, J.B., Dillehay, R.C. and Martin, H.W. (1970) 'Judgments about candidates for psychotherapy: the influence of social class and verbal-insight therapy', *Journal of Health and Social Behavior* 11: 51–8.

Sapir, E. (1929) 'The status of linguistics as a science', *Language* 5: 207–14.

Schafer, R. (1976) *A New Language for Psychoanalysis*, New Haven: Yale University Press.

Shands, H.C. and Meltzer, J.D. (1973) *Language and Psychiatry*, The Hague: Mouton.

Shweder, R.A. and Bourne, E.G. (1984) 'Does the concept of the person vary cross-culturally?', in A.J. Marsella and G.M. White (eds) *Cultural Conceptions of Mental Health and Therapy*, Dordrecht: Reidel.

Sontag, S. (1979) *Illness as Metaphor*, London: Allen Lane.

Szasz, T. (1961) *The Myth of Mental Illness*, New York: Harper & Row.

Titunik, I.R. (1973) 'The formal method and the sociological method (M.M. Baxtin, P.N. Medvedev, V.N. Volosinov) in Russian theory and study of literature', Appendix II in V.N. Volosinov, *Marxism and the Philosophy of Language*, New York: Seminar Press.

Volosinov, V.N. (1973) *Marxism and the Philosophy of Language*, New York: Seminar Press.

Volosinov, V.N. (1976) *Freudianism: A Marxist Critique*, London: Academic Press.

Waissman, F. (1968) *How I See Philosophy*, London: Macmillan.

Weissman, M.M. and Myers, J.K. (1978) 'Rates and risks of depressive disorders in a U.S. suburban community', *Acta Psychiatrica Scandinavica* 57: 219–31.

Whorf, B.L. (1956) *Language, Thought and Reality: Selected Writings of Benjamin Lee Whorf*, New York: Wiley.

Wortman, C.B. and Dunkel-Schetter, C. (1979) 'Interpersonal relationships and cancer: a theoretical analysis', *Journal of Social Issues* 35: 120–55.

Wright, P. and Treacher, A. (1982) 'Introduction', in P. Wright and A. Treacher (eds) *The Problem of Medical Knowledge: Examining the Social Construction of Medicine*, Edinburgh: Edinburgh University Press.

3 Attitude of mind as a means of resisting illness

Kristian Pollock

In recent years there has been increasing interest in lay ideas of health and illness in industrial societies, and the influence of such ideas on preventive health- and illness-related behaviour. To date, only a limited number of studies have been carried out in this area. Many of these have been small and exploratory in nature and have varied in terms of time, location, sample populations and research aims and perspectives. Consequently, it is difficult to undertake any systematic comparison of findings, or to be confident about identifying which ideas are the most important and general in their distribution, or associated with specific groups within the population.

Nevertheless, throughout the available literature, and especially the quoted extracts from interviews with respondents, there is a striking similarity of themes recurring. Several American studies (Zola 1973; (Twaddle 1974; Zborowski 1952) have pointed to ethnic differences in both ideas and behaviour relating to health and illness. However, findings relating to the American 'WASP' population (Twaddle 1974; Baumann 1961; Crawford 1984), to France (Herzlich 1973) and to Britain (Pill and Stott 1982, 1985; Blaxter 1983, 1990; Blaxter and Paterson 1982; Cornwell 1984; Calnan 1987; Pollock 1984; Locker 1981; Williams 1983) suggest a number of intriguing similarities. The majority of respondents surveyed considered their health to be good or very good. At the same time, they acknowledged that for much, if not all of the time, they experienced symptoms of some kind, involving variable degrees of discomfort and disability (see also Wadsworth *et al.* 1971; Hannay 1979; Cartwright and Anderson 1981). It is clear that health is not necessarily or even predominantly identified with the absence of illness, but often defined in functional terms, as the ability to carry out normal everyday tasks and activities. Ill-health is frequently demonstrated by inactivity (e.g. going to bed or staying off work). The relatively low standards or expectations which most people appear to have concerning their health seems to be related to this predominantly functional definition of health. At the same time, people appear to be strongly committed to possessing good health, and are reluctant to acknowledge that it is impaired. This partly explains the sometimes glaring contradictions between respondents' assessments of their own state of health and their actual level of functioning. Apart from its intrinsic desirablity, this commitment to good health stems from its being bound up with ideological and moral concerns. Health is one expression of a person's character or integrity, and is a prerequisite for much of the competence and autonomy which underpins success and achievement in industrial society (Parsons 1972; Crawford 1984). Popular conceptions of health are infused with values which directly reflect those of the dominant ideology of industrial society.

Control of health is one direct expression of control of the self (Crawford 1984). At the same time, as several studies suggest (Herzlich 1973; Pollock 1984; Blaxter and Paterson 1982; Blaxter 1990), the attribution of personal responsibility for health and illness is quite subtle and complex. People are prepared to assume some responsibility for their general health, and in so doing to believe they have some capacity to influence their susceptibility to routine everyday illnesses, such as colds and 'flu. On the other hand, it is evident from a number of the studies cited that most people adopt a predominantly fatalistic attitude to more serious disorders, such as cancer or heart disease. These illnesses are a manifestation of misfortune: they just happen. Herzlich (1973) characterized this idea in terms of the distinction between self as the 'source of health' and other as the 'bringer of illness'. It seems that people are willing to assume some responsibility for good health, but not for serious illness.

Throughout the literature there has also been a more than passing reference to the importance of ideas about 'attitude of mind' or 'mind over matter'. These are directly related to ideas about personal responsibility for, and control over, health and illness. In my own research into concepts of health and illness among families in Nottingham, such ideas were widespread and significant. In what follows I describe its various applications as applied to 'general health' and 'particular illness' and the ways in which these differ in relation to serious physical and mental disorders.

BACKGROUND TO THE STUDY

Fieldwork was carried out in Nottingham between July 1979 and September 1980. Three groups of families were involved. In the first of these one member of each family was affected by multiple sclerosis (MS), in the second, by schizophrenia. The third group was made up of relatively 'healthy' families unaffected by serious physical or mental illness. My research focused on the role of knowledge about health and illness as a resource affecting the ability of families to adjust to serious illness. A good deal of background information was collected about each of the 105 families involved in the study. Initial (Family) interviews covered family structure and organization, social and kinship networks, respondents' accounts of the patient's illness and the family's contact with the health and social services. A total of 114 representatives from 78 families also participated in a further (Health) interview which explored ideas about health and illness. This interview included a detailed exploration of images and beliefs concerning six specific illnesses: nervous breakdown, multiple sclerosis, schizophrenia, cancer, heart attack and stroke. Face-to-face contact with each family ranged from one to thirty hours, with averages of four hours for the Family interview and three hours for the Health interview. Additional sources of data included case notes and other research data relating to a number of schizophrenia patients,[1] and my informal involvement with the local branches of the relevant self-help groups CRACK MS (the self-help section of the MS Society) and the National Schizophrenia Fellowship. Although the Health interview was the single most important source of information about ideas relating to attitude of mind, I have taken account of relevant material scattered throughout all the various sources of data to which I had access.

Respondents varied in age and socioeconomic background, though the majority (73 per cent of Health interview respondents) belonged to social classes 2 and 3. Sixty per cent were women. Of the 114 respondents who took part in the Health interview, 48 belonged to the MS group, 33 to the schizophrenia group and 33 to the ordinary group. Further details concerning data collection and the composition of the different illness groups are given in Pollock (1984).

ATTITUDE OF MIND

Most respondents considered that body and mind exerted a reciprocal influence insofar as mental attitude was thought to influence both susceptibility to illness and its outcome, while a sick body could also produce illness in the mind. In most cases this influence was not thought to be symmetrical. A much greater emphasis was placed on the power of the mind to influence bodily processes and determine the individual's state of health than the converse. Statements referring to the importance of 'attitude of mind' occurred frequently in a variety of contexts throughout the interviews and testified to the significance which many respondents attached to the assumed ability of 'mind' to control 'matter'. This idea was expressed by 87 per cent (N = 86) of respondents, with varying degrees of emphasis.[2] Twenty-five per cent of respondents strongly articulated the importance of attitude of mind throughout the interviews. Over half of these were MS sufferers or their spouses. There was a consistent tendency for MS respondents to place the greatest emphasis, and ordinary respondents the least emphasis, on the importance of attitude of mind, with the schizophrenia group coming in between the other two. Only 13 respondents thought there was little or no relationship between attitude of mind and health. I discuss later on the ways in which respondents directly affected by illness, particularly physical illness, made greater use of these ideas about attitude of mind.

Respondents varied in the strength of their opinions about the importance of attitude of mind in determining health, but mind was considered to be the most vital aspect of the person. The body, as mere 'matter' was relegated to a position of secondary significance. To the extent that the body was thought to be controlled by the mind it could also be viewed as an expression of strength of will.

> 'The mind is the same to all people. It is put there to control one's life, to control and guide physical effort, so everyone has the ability to do this ... it depends whether or not they cultivate it a lot. Those who fall by the wayside just haven't got that strong base.'

The mind is supposed to control the person through an exercise of will, and is thus a manifestation of his humanity. This idea is forcefully expressed in the following statement from a man who was severely disabled by MS.

> 'The pain I've got I can live with. The only thing I've got to cleave to is my mind. A man's nowt without his mind .... If a man's loony, in a mental institution ... that's what life's all about, thinking, being able to work things out, big problems, little problems. That's the only thing I've got to cling to now, with my body going the way it has, is saying what's what in my family. If you've no mind, you're nowt, you're just not there .... That's what separates us from the animals: a brain. You're as good as dead if you ain't got a mind. You're dead, aren't you? With sanity you've got everything. You miss the running about and the normal things of life .... At least I can think.'

Although dependent on the brain, by means of which it functions, mind is at the same time separate from it, an expression of a 'higher' principle.

> 'Mind is the thought cells which are controlled by a higher thing, which is you, and that is the will.'

However, a consequence of the very close relationship between the brain and the mind is that when the brain is damaged the basis of the will is also impaired, so that 'mind over matter' can no longer be applied. For this reason it was recognized that in the case of certain illnesses such as stroke or schizophrenia it was difficult, if not impossible, for recovery to occur.

Recovery depended on the ability of the sick person to want to get better and to actively participate in his or her cure. If there was no such organic impediment inhibiting recovery then individuals were thought to be capable of helping themselves to get better, and it was felt to be appropriate and desirable that they should do so. Failure to cooperate in the process of recovery was attributed to either a lack of motivation or a defective will. Both of these were generally taken to be indicative of a 'weak' person. Attitudes towards such inadequates ranged from the tolerantly sympathetic (some people simply can't help being weaker than others) to the overtly critical (anyone could help themselves through a greater effort of will and ought to do so). In most cases the question of motivation was regarded as more or less a matter of individual choice. It was up to the people concerned whether or not they wanted to get better: they were not obliged to do so. If they did not, although people might think less of them as a result, they were not thought to have committed any kind of moral transgression.

Attitude of mind in relation to general health

'General' health related primarily to the absence of minor complaints. It was the taken-for-granted norm. Attitude of mind was thought relevant here both insofar as it could strengthen resistance to illnesses such as colds, minor infections, aches and pains, etc., and could also determine the individual's reaction to these if and when he was afflicted. People could worry unreasonably about their health, and they could worry themselves into either thinking they had ailments when in fact they did not, or also, if they were persistent, into actually developing illnesses unnecessarily. Statements such as the following were common.

> 'People can worry too much about health. Generally you get the health you deserve. If you think you're going to be healthy then you will be .... '

> 'You can make yourself healthy or you can make yourself unhealthy. You can work for or against health. It's in the mind.'

> 'For me it's all in the mind. A lot of illness is all in the mind.'

Having got an illness of some kind, the approved reaction was not to make a meal of it, but as far as possible to ignore and underplay the difficulties and discomforts it involved. Such a disregard of its effects, allied with sufficient determination to send it speedily on its way, would assist in a rapid recovery.

> 'If you think, "Oh, well, I'll get over this", then you will.'

> 'I imagine it's up to the person ... I mean, if you let yourself sort of ... suffer, I suppose you'll suffer more than if you say, "Oh, I'm not having

> this, I'm going to shake it off". Some people are stronger-minded than others.'

Thus, as far as everyday complaints were concerned, the appropriate reaction, at least in theory, was 'not to give in' but to 'rise above them'. In effect, it was often seen to be one's 'attitude' that determined how much one allowed oneself to suffer from the relatively trivial or temporary disorders that come within the scope of general health.

Attitude of mind in relation to physical illness

Most people did not think that attitude of mind had much, if any, effect on preventing serious illness. Not much could be done to avoid these, and protective measures were usually thought to involve behaviour rather than will-power. However, attitude of mind in relation to physical illness was thought to be important in two ways. It could determine the kind of recovery that was made and even, indeed, whether recovery was achieved at all.

> 'The doctors can only fight a losing battle if there is no will to live.'

> 'Some people say, "Oh, I wish they'd tell me [if I had cancer]", but I don't think people really want to know, deep down. I think it's better they don't know. If they're never really sure then there's always a bit of hope. But if you say "You've got cancer", I think they want to give up, a lot of people, you know. But I think your state of mind can make it better or worse again. My father nearly died of it [cancer] and the doctor was so surprised that he managed to survive, which he did, and that was 30 years ago he had that, and there wasn't as much of a chance then as today, perhaps. But he's got a great constitution and a will to live, you see, and there's your difference, from one who hasn't got much will, or ... wants to give up.'

The conviction that people can, at least in certain circumstances, literally will themselves to live or die is striking, and was not uncommon. A less drastic, but probably more significant idea is that a person's attitude of mind is important in determining how he or she reacts to an illness that is chronic or permanently disabling.

> 'There is a lot of determination in how you react to illness. The attitude you adopt is very important, perhaps the most important thing.'

> 'A lot of it is up to yourself, if you have strong willpower. This enables a person to come to terms with what they've got, it can't prevent things from happening in the first place. The best reaction is, you just think it isn't there.'

The normative reaction is to make light of one's affliction, to carry on as usual, and as far as possible to adopt the behaviour appropriate to a healthy person. While this type of reaction may have some adaptive value for the individual sufferer, it is likely that its greatest significance lies in facilitating the way in which the healthy accommodate the disabled. As Freidson (1970) notes, in contrast to acute illnesses, chronic disabilities are awarded permanent legitimation. At the same time, this is conditional on sufferers making an effort to 'improve' themselves, and make themselves socially acceptable by minimizing the demands he makes on other people. In other words, social stereotypes concerning the appropriate reactions to long-term and incurable illness limit the amount of 'deviant' behaviour which is tolerated among the chronically ill.

From the observations made during this study, my impression is that these ideas about the appropriate way to react to serious physical illness tend to be reinforced by workers in the volunatry, welfare and professional health services. Failure to conform to the appropriate stereotype is likely to meet with hostility and intolerance on the part of both professionals and laymen concerned with the sufferer. Adherence to it may provide many sufferers with a positive and satisfying model around which to orient their behaviour. Alternatively, the pressure to conform can make heavy demands on individual resilience and fortitude, and this may become burdensome to those unable or unwilling to comply.

Respondents' representations about 'attitude of mind' and its effects depict an ideal rather than an often realized, or even realizable, state of affairs. People varied in the extent to which their own behaviour approximated to it. Nevertheless, I was impressed by the conviction with which a number of respondents had apparently mastered the practice of correct attitude of mind, as well as the accompanying rhetoric. On the other hand, precisely because acceptance of the desirability of adopting such an attitude in response to illness was so widespread, there was a tendency to pay lip-service to a principle which, consciously or otherwise, people did not actually practice. This does not in any way diminish the significance of attitude of mind as a social representation, though it does have interesting implications for studies which rely on stereotyped attitude testing for their results.

Attitude of mind in relation to mental illness

It is in relation to mental illness that the importance of attitude of mind was most frequently and strongly stated. In contrast to physical illness, mental illness was often thought to be unnecessary, and avoidable through sufficient effort of will. A few respondents maintained that conditions such as 'nervous breakdown' and 'depression' were not so much 'illnesses' as 'states of mind', and, therefore, controllable wholly through adoption of the right 'attitude of mind'.

> 'To be quite honest, I don't class it as an illness ... because people can get over it if they try. ... It's all a matter of determination.'

> 'Depression is just a state of mind. You can do something about that yourself ... . Nervous breakdown. You can fight yourself out of a nervous breakdown.'

Most people did regard conditions such as nervous breakdown and depression as 'illness', though of a rather anomalous kind. One of the ways in which mental and physical illness were contrasted was in terms of the 'invisibility' of mental illness. Since there is 'nothing to show for it' the suspicion arises that mental illness may be in some way less 'substantial' than physical illness, and in any particular case, less 'genuine'. The legitimacy of adopting the sick role for mental illness is likely to be much more problematic than for most kinds of physical illness.

Serious physical illness was regarded as misfortune which the individual had little power to prevent. Even where personal negligence or foolishness may have contributed to its onset, physical illness was not thought to be avoidable through an effort of will. Nor was it something the individual wanted to happen to him. Central to the concept of 'illness', for which physical illness served as a paradigm, was the idea that it was involuntary and unwelcome. Because most serious illnesses were not thought to be easily preventable, people were not held responsible for them. However, a recurrent theme concerning mental illness was that it may be motivated. This was clearly related to the widespread suspicion attached to such disorders. Insofar as it was something the individual had the power to control, it was also something for which he or she could be held responsible.

Nervous breakdown was often thought to result from an individual having 'given in', or failing to 'get a grip on himself'. It was a form of 'escape', a refusal to face up to life's problems and difficulties.

> 'A nervous breakdown is an unconscious psychological get-out of life's problems.'

It was often regarded as an expression of personal weakness, a failure to exert sufficient will-power and determination.

> 'If someone is subject to a breakdown, then somewhere along the line they have lost their own will. If they had a strong will then they wouldn't have allowed it to happen. When they get on a psychiatrist's couch they are made to realize their own foolishness and that this caused it and then they can fully recover.'

There is a sense in which people were thought, if not exactly to 'will' themselves into a breakdown, then to have one as a result of not wanting strongly enough to prevent it. For some respondents, whether or not an individual reacted to circumstances by having a breakdown, or resisting the pressures to do so, was largely a matter of choice.

> 'You see, I've nerves ... and I've got to admit that I could afford to have one according to my doctor, but I didn't because I didn't want one ... .'

> 'You've got to take your life in your hands. You haven't got to have one. I got depressed once and the doctor told me that I didn't have time to have a breakdown, with two kids to care for. Anyone could have one, I suppose ... s'pose it is bad, but you've got to be firm with yourself ... . I haven't got time for nerves. If I'm tense ... I get into something, do the housework, or the washing. Keep myself active, instead of sitting and worrying, feeling sorry for myself.'

The idea that a breakdown was indicative of personal weakness was often associated with the idea that it was always, or usually, a certain 'type' of person who was susceptible. Alternatively, some respondents felt that there was a certain 'type' of person, themselves usually included, who would never have a breakdown under any circumstances.

> 'I can't see anyone like myself ever having a nervous breakdown, or allowing it to happen. Never to me. I'm not that type of person.'

> 'If you've got a ... oh, dear, how can I put it? ... Some people have a strong will, strong mind, don't they? Some are born with a ... not so strong that way, it seems, within them. It's the type of person you are, more susceptible. When you're strong-minded, I think it's less inclined for it to happen. I think you might get a physical disease perhaps, if illness strikes, but ... it just depends ... very sensitive people I think would be prone to get it, over-sensitive, or, in the case of my husband, he was always a bit immature, and this need of security, I *think* is part of his trouble.'

Nervous breakdown clearly had pejorative connotations for many respondents. It was thought to be an expression of personal weakness, often in a foolish, immature, inadequate personality. Only a small number of respondents admitted to being the 'kind of person' who suffered from 'nerves' or was likely to have a breakdown. With the exception of schizophrenia and MS, which were both illnesses often associated with a genetic or hereditary cause, nervous breakdown was the only illness which some respondents were prepared to say they were sure they would never get.

Regardless of the extent to which susceptibility to a nervous breakdown was thought to result from a person's strength of character or innate susceptibility, 'stress ' was thought by all respondents to precipitate the illness, if it did not cause it outright. It was widely acknowledged that in extraordinarily difficult or stressful circumstances anyone could have a breakdown. Many people were prepared to accept that in some cases, albeit extreme ones, there were 'reasonable grounds' for someone to break down. In this case the general assumption concerning personal responsibility for the illness was largely overriden. Although they might concede that in the end everyone did have a 'breaking point', respondents often acknowledged this grudgingly, and only when pressed.

Many people seemed to feel that although a nervous breakdown could be a reasonable and legitimate response to experiences of an intensely traumatic nature, in practice it was not exposure to this kind of situation which caused the majority of breakdowns.

> 'They're things you can, I won't say fight against, but you can get over them. They're not crippling. I don't have any fear of them. You can control them, and often it is a certain type of person who gets them. Yes, they are avoidable – though if you have a terrible run of bad luck, with many bereavements and so on, then maybe anyone would have a breakdown. But the self-pitying type of breakdown, that's another matter altogether.'

> 'I think you've got to be quite a weak person to get a nervous breakdown, and this can often be self-induced. I don't let things worry me, so I would never have one .... Sometimes, if everything went bad people could be more likely to have a breakdown, but some people never would, whatever happened, because they just don't react that way. ... Some people are weaker than others, but I feel that often people could help themselves and prevent themselves from having a breakdown. I know a lot of people wouldn't agree with that.'

It is interesting that several schizophrenia patients who had made a good recovery from what they thought had been a nervous breakdown or depression used a similar framework to interpret their experience. They said their illness had been a response to an intensely stressful period in their lives, and could never happen again. They felt their own determination to 'pull themselves out of it' had played a large part in their subsequent recovery. In fact, from an observer's point of view, there was little to account for why these respondents should have become ill at one particular point in their lives rather than a number of others. In addition, it was clear that each of them had received a fairly prolonged and intensive course of treatment, though the effects of this tended to be underplayed in their accounts of their illness and their own reactions to it.

Irrespective of the reasons which caused people to become ill in the first place, once someone suffered a nervous breakdown or depression, they were expected to help themselves to get better. In this respect, mental and physical illness were thought to be similar. Recovery depended on the active participation of the patient, and would be inhibited or prevented from taking place if the patient did not actively want to get better.

> 'What you make yourself you can mend yourself.'

> 'The patient has got to pull himself through. The doctors can only do so much. If the patient doesn't want to come back, you've had it. People do recover, but it's not a hundred per cent foolproof cure. You'll be cured if you want to be cured. Some people are just the type who haven't got the fight in them. Other people just can't cope with a particular crisis but can pull themselves out of it.'

A third of all respondents felt that it was usual for people to make a more or less complete recovery from a nervous breakdown. This was generally thought to be achieved through the combination of medical treatment and the patient's own efforts to help him- or herself. Some respondents commented on a further complication attaching to nervous breakdown. Recovery from all forms of illness required the active cooperation of the patient. However, in the case of mental illness it was the will itself which was 'diseased' and often because of this patients were unable to help themselves, making recovery much more difficult and protracted, if not ultimately impossible.

> 'If you're ill, you've got to have the mental ability to turn around and get better. But in mental illness the mind's gone, so it is much harder to recover. Patients can help themselves to a certain extent with the help of the doctors, but they have got to accept that they are ill first.'

This idea, that it was difficult for mentally ill patients to help themselves towards recovery, was a minority view. A much more frequently expressed idea was that the patient was at least partially responsible for his or her own recovery. Consequently, when they failed to get better, this was likely to be regarded as their own fault. Either they did not really want to get better, or they had not tried hard enough. In the first case they were likely to be suspected of malingering, in the second of being weak and spineless.

I have outlined some of the principal themes which occurred during discussions of respondents' ideas about mental illness. There was considerable variation in the ways these were combined and the strength of opinions held by different respondents. For example, some people emphasized the individual's responsibility for becoming mentally ill, and for making a recovery. Others stressed the scope for personal intervention in relation to only one of these stages. Some respondents said that a person could not do anything to prevent a breakdown in the face of circumstances that completely overpowered him, but he could and should help himself to recover from it. Others felt that it was easier to avoid a breakdown in the first place, through adopting an appropriate attitude of mind, than it was to participate in a recovery, because by that time it was too late, the mind had 'gone', and so on. Many respondents clearly thought that to have had a breakdown cast a slur on a person's character and placed his or her integrity in doubt. I think it is this association of breakdown with weakness and loss of control that underlies much of the stigma that still attaches to it. Respondents varied in the sympathy or tolerance they felt for people affected by mental illness. Many adopted a fairly neutral attitude. Nevertheless, I was surprised by the number of people who expressed overt hostility and criticism of the mentally ill, and by the readiness with which they were prepared to subject them to censure.

Attitude of mind in relation to multiple sclerosis

Although respondents in both the ordinary and schizophrenia groups rarely mentioned the idea that attitude of mind could be effectively applied against MS, it was characteristic of MS sufferers that they did do so. In this respect sufferers tended to conform to the general stereotype concerning the appropriate form of response to serious physical illness. That this was often not a spontaneous reaction is indicated in the accounts of sufferers who described the process of adjustment following disclosure of the diagnosis of MS, and their struggle to come to terms with the knowledge that they were affected by a long-term and chronically disabling illness. For example, one sufferer recalled the devastation he felt when he learned he had MS: 'I thought it was like the black plague'. Later on he met other sufferers and talking to them helped him adjust to his illness. Then he thought:

> 'Come on, get a hold of yourself, mate. You're not dead yet. You have a certain span of life, and you have to make the best of it. But make sure you don't become a cabbage.'

Another respondent said he had been shocked by the diagnosis of MS, but subsequently he came to terms with it.

> 'Well, it's there. Everyone said, "Well, it's only a matter of determination". You have to help yourself.'

As these examples suggest, sufferers were often helped and encouraged by other people to adopt 'attitude of mind' as a means of resisting the illness. Experienced sufferers provided the newly diagnosed with a model of how to react to the illness and encouraged them to adopt it. This process was most strikingly demonstrated within the CRACK group, the self-help division of the MS society (discussed more fully in Pollock 1984). However, encouraging the sufferer to adopt an appropriate attitude of mind was also the explicit goal of the social, welfare and voluntary workers with whom I came in contact. In effect, the extent to which a sufferer was regarded as being 'well' or 'poorly' adjusted to his illness was considered largely in terms of his attitude to it, specifically whether he was prepared to 'help himself' through his own determination and will-power, or whether he preferred to 'give in', and adopt a passive, negative, self-pitying attitude. Instances of the latter were rare, which I found surprising, although the distinction between the well-adjusted active sufferer and the poorly adjusted passive sufferer was emphasized very frequently.

The majority of MS sufferers accepted the desirability of adopting a positive attitude of mind towards their illness. This was one of the basic components of 'self-help' which was also widely favoured and practised.[3] This does not mean that these sufferers were all at once, or for all time, provided with a satisfying and effective means of resisting their illness and reducing the threat it posed for them. The model of attitude of mind represented an ideal, to which individual sufferers approximated as best they could. Attitude of mind could not eliminate the fear, bitterness, depression or insecurity that sufferers experienced in relation to their illness, especially during periods of relapse. No doubt there were discrepancies between the public face of many sufferers, presented in terms of bravado, self-reliance and determination, and their private fears and insecurities. Nevertheless, the model did serve as a point of reference and a guide for action. By declaring a commitment to a positive attitude of mind sufferers win respect and approval from their family and friends, other sufferers, and also workers from the various services with whom they come in contact. At the same time, they are provided with a means of boosting their own confidence and self-esteem. There is no doubt that a number of sufferers had successfuly internalized the principles of attitude of mind, the practice of which had become an important part of their identity. In this way the commitment to attitude of mind can be seen to shape the sufferer's behaviour and assist in the process of adjustment to their illness. It also facilitates the process of adjustment of the able-bodied towards the disabled.

Attitude of mind in relation to schizophrenia

With very few exceptions respondents did not regard attitude of mind as relevant to schizophrenia. Schizophrenia was commonly thought to involve some kind of intrinsic defect or impairment. People were 'born' with it, and it could not be prevented or cured. Attitude of mind could not be applied because the basis of the will was thought to have been destroyed. One of the most salient and disturbing facts about schizophrenia was that it was thought to involve absolute loss of control. The individual was not held responsible for his or her illness, and was not thought capable of doing anything to help him- or herself recover from it.

'FIGHTING' ILLNESS

The principle embodied in attitude of mind is clearly articulated in the metaphor of 'fighting' illness, references to which recur frequently throughout the literature (e.g. Herzlich 1973; Blaxter and Paterson 1982; Pill and Stott 1982, 1985; Williams 1983; Crawford 1984; Calnan 1987). This was felt to be an appropriate response, regardless of whether or not respondents had themselves been directly confronted with serious illness.

> 'Some people are capable of overcoming a lot of illness. You can give in a lot to illness and make it worse. There is definitely a lot of illness you can fight, though I don't believe it is a hundred per cent mind over matter. On the other hand the reverse is extremely true, and some people can induce illness and magnify things to a great extent.'

The ability to 'fight' is generally assumed to vary between individuals. Its application in relation to illness is thought to be one manifestation of a more general aspect of the person, expressive of a characteristic manner of dealing with the world.

> 'I mean, if you're born to be a fighter, you'll probably always be a fighter to the end. But if you succumb to these things, well ... .'

A third of all respondents (N=38) said that one should respond to illness by 'fighting' it, though there were differences in the emphasis placed on this idea, and the contexts in which it was applied. As with attitude of mind, the idea that one can fight illness was most commonly encountered among respondents from both the sick groups, who mentioned it twice as often as ordinary respondents. It was most clearly emphasized and articulated by respondents suffering from MS.

Fighting multiple sclerosis

The importance of adopting a positive attitude, trying to help oneself as much as possible, and what this could achieve even in the face of severe physical disability, was stressed over and over again, not just by individual respondents, but also in CRACK group meetings and in various publications put out by the MS Society, CRACK and ARMS (Action and Research into

Multiple Sclerosis, another self-help organization concerned with MS). This position was echoed by workers from the voluntary, welfare and medical services. Within all these groups the same distinction between two kinds of sufferer was frequently encountered. 'Active' sufferers resisted their illness and did everything they could to help themselves and overcome the difficulties resulting from it. 'Passive' sufferers 'gave in' to their illness, being content to let other people do for them things they could do for themselves, while they wallowed in apathy and self-pity. The difference between these two categories of sufferers was often characterized in terms of whether or not they were prepared to 'fight' MS.

It was typical of many CRACK members, as well as a number of MS sufferers outside the sphere of CRACK who were also committed to the practice of self-help, that they chose to engage the enemy in the domain of the body as well as the mind. Indeed, it may be that this predilection for action is one of the things that attracts individual sufferers to become involved with groups like CRACK. However, it was not necessary to engage in concrete, practical action in order to 'fight' the illness effectively. Essentially, MS is fought by refusing to give in to it, regardless of whether the battle is extended into the field of the corporeal or confined within the mind and spirit of the sufferer, whose most powerful weapon is constituted in the exercise of will. This means of conceptualizing an appropriate and desirable strategy for dealing with the illness renders it accessible both to the severely disabled as well as the relatively able-bodied sufferer. Different individuals might disagree about how much control it was possible to achieve over the illness through the practice of self-help. Circumstances might force a revision of a sufferer's assessment of what could be achieved by attitude of mind. No matter how severely disabled he or she might become, however, and even when it was recognized that it was no longer possible to bring about any material improvement in his physical health, it was still possible to believe in the positive effects resulting from the practice of attitude of mind, as well as the desirability of adopting this kind of reaction for its own sake.

I do not mean to suggest that because many MS sufferers had ready access to a strategy for coping with the illness, encapsulated within the fighting metaphor, it was an easy one to adopt, or because reactions such as fear, depression and hopelessness were formally disallowed in the model, that individual sufferers did not sometimes succumb to them. The ideology of self-help, of fighting MS, provided sufferers with a rhetoric of optimism and a guide to conduct rather than a description of reality. Nevertheless, there were tangible benefits to be gained from the adoption of the self-help model of MS. The value of this was highlighted both by observation of cases of MS where sufferers either did not have access to this, or could not accept or make use of it, and also of the families of the schizophrenia patients, who lacked any such tool for the conceptualization and management of their illness.

Self-help oriented MS sufferers often had a clearly articulated awareness of their own strength of character. This did not exactly express itself in a sense of superiority over other 'normal' people, but it seemed to be one way in which such respondents tended to set themselves off against others. This was most clearly revealed in their evaluation of 'strength' and 'weakness' in relation to susceptibility to ill-health, which I have discussed above. Respondents from the MS group, especially sufferers, tended to adopt a rather harsher and more intolerant attitude towards people suffering from mental illness than was true of those from the other two groups. Self-help oriented sufferers very commonly also set themselves off from other sufferers in similar terms.

The conviction that it was possible to control or contain the illness was always vulnerable to challenge from the negative instances which pointed to the contrary. I think this may be one reason for the strength and prevalence of the conviction that many MS sufferers are not willing to fight, and that it is their inability or unwillingness to adequately resist the illness that accounts for the severity of their disability. Thus, if it was possible to help oneself to better health, the converse was also implied. There was the suspicion that cases of severe disability were, or could be, the result of failure to do so, the consequence, once again, of a defective or inadequate will. This explanation of why extreme disability happened to other people and not oneself enabled sufferers to construct a plausible defence against the possibility that the same fate might one day befall themselves. This was a way of thinking about things in general, because no sufferer could discount the possibility that the illness could move with great speed and devastation, regardless of anything he could do to prevent it. The unpredictability of the illness and the uniqueness of each case were also central tenets within the corpus of knowledge about MS. This uncertainty worked both ways, however, since it also enabled more severely disabled sufferers to hope that sudden improvement and drastic remissions could occur. These were known to happen occasionally.

The inability to 'fight' schizophrenia

The notion of 'fighting' illness has no relevance to schizophrenia. I have commented on the consistency with which respondents from all three groups regarded this as an illness which the individual was powerless to control. Among respondents not directly affected by it, schizophrenia was often thought to result from some kind of intrinsic defect of the person, and commonly assumed to be inherited. The sufferer was not held responsible for the illness, or thought capable of participating in recovery from it. In this context, the only 'informed' respondents were the small group of relatives and a few patients who were aware of the diagnosis of schizophrenia. The majority had assumed, or sometimes been told that the patient had suffered a 'nervous breakdown'. Most 'informed' relatives seemed to have achieved a fairly good understanding and tolerance of the patient's illness. Although a few entertained certain suspicions, these relatives generally accepted that the patient's illness rendered him unable to help himself, even if they considered this to be an appropriate course of action in relation to other kinds of sickness.

Most of those affected by MS saw it as something which happens to a person, but does not threaten the viability or integrity of the personality. Unlike schizophrenia, MS never becomes a fundamental attribute of the person. We do not speak of a 'multiple sclerotic' as we do of a 'schizophrenic'. Schizophrenia often seems to be experienced by patients and perceived by their relatives as an invasive force, completely taking over the person, so that he becomes something other than what he was. This transmutation of the person is not easily reversible. Even after acute episodes of the illness are over, this demonstration of the capacity for madness, once manifest, leaves the suspicion that it may recur. It brings with it the realization that there is something fundamentally different about the individual so affected. He or she will rarely be perceived in the same way again. In cases of chronic schizophrenia the evidence of a transformed character is clear enough, and often distressingly permanent.

The most disturbing and dreaded aspect of both MS and schizophrenia is loss of control, in the one case of the body, and in the other of the mind. With MS, however – and this is a feature stressed particularly within the ideology of self-help – regardless of the physical degeneration which may occur, the mind not only remains intact, but also retains the potentiality for further development. There is a sense in which one may become more of a person than one was before. With schizophrenia, on the other hand, one can only become less, because central to the illness is the fragmentation of the mind, the disintegration of the will which, as we have seen, is often felt to be the most powerful expression of humanity. Schizophrenic patients often simply cannot help themselves, which makes it very hard for their family or anyone else to help them either. MS sufferers can separate themselves from their illness, objectify it, and turn it into an enemy they can fight, primarily through the exercise of their own determination and will-power. Schizophrenia patients cannot externalize their affliction in this way, and lack the means to offer any such resistance to it.

Very few respondents thought it possible to recover from either MS or schizophrenia. Both illnesses were widely regarded as catastrophic. Nevertheless, there were important differences between the ways in which these illnesses were perceived. These differences had very real consequences for the ways in which those afflicted by them were able to respond. The self-help model of MS, with its emphasis on the power of 'attitude of mind' and the ability of the individual sufferer to 'fight' his illness, assumes that he is not merely a helpless victim, but can achieve a good deal through his or her own effort and motivation. In addition, it provides a concrete plan of action which can at least help them, and at best wholly enable them, to minimize his or her disability. The model offers a means of encouraging confidence and hope for a feasible future. This view of the illness insists that having MS does not mean that the sufferer is invariably going to be reduced to a helpless cripple, and attempts to normalize the condition by holding out the possibility of a productive and active life. The self-help model of MS develops certain ideas about culturally appropriate responses to illness, and thus promotes the sufferer's acceptability within the world of the able-bodied. In addition, the distinctive means of conceptualizing the illness as something external to, and other than, oneself, as an 'enemy' to be actively resisted and fought, constitutes a powerful ally in the process of adjustment. This is not available to patients affected by schizophrenia, or to their relatives. Nor is there available any culturally sanctioned or appropriate model in terms of which schizophrenia may be accommodated. Prevailing conceptions of attitude of mind in relation to health and illness work to the advantage of those affected by serious physical disability and disorder, but constitute an additional handicap to patients and relatives attempting to make a viable adjustment to serious mental illnesses, such as schizophrenia.

CONCLUSION

Ideas about attitude of mind in relation to health and illness constitute a specific application of more general and pervasive social representations about appropriate responses to hardship and misfortune. The extent to which popular conceptions of health and illness involve moral judgements about personal integrity and competence is a recurrent theme throughout the literature. A particular interest has been the extent to which people feel they can control their health, or are prepared to assume responsibility for illness. Underlying this has been a practical concern, since it has been assumed that unless people are prepared to accept some responsibility they will not be receptive to the message of health education programmes which emphazise the importance of behavioural change at an individual level in reducing morbidity within the population as a whole (Pill and Stott 1982, 1985). Similarly, a pragmatic justification for the value and relevance of research into lay concepts was that health education could be more effectively targeted, and its success evaluated, once the nature and extent of popular knowledge about health and illness was established. Again, it was assumed that when people became aware of the relationship between health and behaviour they would be sufficiently motivated to adopt a 'healthier' lifestyle. In fact, recent research suggests not only that the relationship between health beliefs and behaviour is rather slight, but also that the contribution of supposedly 'healthy' behaviours to health status is limited, and far outweighed by the effects of socioeconomic status (Blaxter 1990; Davison *et al.* 1991).

The findings of my own and other studies suggest that people believe they have some influence over the quality of their general health, but are reluctant to accept responsibility for illness. Most people adopted a fairly fatalistic attitude to the occurrence of serious physical disorders, which were beyond the reach of personal control or prevention. A more salient issue especially in relation to physical illness is not so much apportioning blame or responsibility, as evaluating the nature of the person through his or her response to it, and in particular, his or her strength of constitution and of mind (Crawford 1984; Blaxter 1990; Blaxter and Paterson 1982; Cornwell 1984; Williams 1983). Despite being largely taken for granted (except in its absence) health is highly valued, and often regarded as a prerequisite for autonomy and personal achievement. Regardless of whether it is considered preventable, illness spoils identity and threatens to diminish the person. It is in this context that the ideas about attitude of mind can be brought into play to offset this threat, and even override it. This was demonstrated by the MS sufferers described above, who stressed the pre-eminence of mind over matter. These ideas were clearly helpful to many sufferers in their effort to fashion a viable response to their illness and the disabilities it imposed. As we have seen, however, the effects of such constructs were to compound the disadvantages and stigmatizing effects of mental illness ('nervous breakdown') and 'madness' (schizophrenia).

The findings of recent studies increasingly challenge an earlier assumption that there is little convergence between popular and biomedical models of health and illness. On the one hand, popular interest in medicine and its spectacular technological achievements, and the popularization and widespread dissemination of medical knowledge have produced a well-informed public. Indeed, research by Tuckett and his associates (1985) suggests that it is the patient's ability to undertake extensive and usually accurate interpretive work that determines the relatively successful outcome of most routine medical encounters. On the other hand, and this seems often to have been overlooked, doctors and other health workers are themselves steeped in the same cultural constructs that influence the motivation and understanding of their patients. Indeed, medical culture can hardly avoid being underpinned by the prevailing social representations which it also helps to shape. The ideological component of medical activity can easily be concealed under the mantle of 'science' and the authority this bestows. There is a reciprocal and reflexive interaction between medical and social constructs. Ideas deriving from either the popular or medical sectors are developed within the framework of the authority and supposed objectivity of scientific research, fed back into society, and re-examined in the course of further research development. In an earlier article I have illustrated this process with reference to the stress discourse (Pollock 1988). I have already commented on the way in which health and social workers seemed to evaluate patients' adjustment to illness and disability in the same way as the sufferers themselves, and specifically with reference to the individual's willingness to resist and 'fight' illness. Current interest in 'psychogenic' illness seems to incorporate the development and application of ideas about attitude of mind and to extend these in a rather sinister fashion. In the 'scientific' rather than the popular domain there has been a trend towards locating individual susceptibility to illness in features of personality. Coronary heart disease and cancer have been singled out for particular attention in this regard (Pollock 1988). Sontag (1979) has argued eloquently that attempts to psychologize illness in this way provide an accurate means of charting areas of medical ignorance and impotence. As she notes, particularly with reference to TB, once an illness is subject to effective control and treatment, psychosomatic theories of causation are rendered redundant and quickly abandoned. Contemporary efforts to link personality and illness are disturbing because they redefine the source of illness as the self rather than biology or chance or socio-economic circumstances. This is to dissolve the existing culturally defined barrier between physical and mental illness and ultimately to reduce the individual's ability to resist illness or adjust to disability in terms of the cultural constructs described above. As was illustrated by the MS sufferers, the 'self' is the means through which one 'fights' illness. On the other hand, when the self itself is flawed or inadequate, one cannot effectively fight, as was the case with those suffering from madness (schizophrenia) or, to a lesser extent, mental illness (nervous breakdown). Moreover, this idea of the individual as the source of his or her own illness is particularly damaging to his or her self-esteem, and public evaluation. So far, as the results of available studies indicate, popular opinion has resisted or remained unaware of the attempt to link specific disorders with personality traits, with most people expressing a broadly fatalistic outlook regarding the genesis of serious illness. It remains to be seen whether such ideas gain wider social currency. From a sociological standpoint, I find the attempt to psychologize illness subversive insofar as it reinforces the trend towards the individualization of illness, and the medical and political commitment to health as a matter of personal rather than social responsibility.

NOTES

1 These were included in an international investigation of the social determinants of outcome of schizophrenia carried out by the World Health Organization (1973, 1975, 1979). Nottingham was one of the study's research centres.

2 There was some variation in the response base to some of the questions asked in the Health Interview, i.e. N does not always equal 114. This was largely because of the exploratory nature of the first interviews, most of which were carried out with MS respondents. A number of additional questions were subsequently incorporated into the interview schedule in response to ideas which emerged during these initial discussions. In addition, some responses were subsequently judged to be inadequate or too ambiguous to allow accurate coding. Occasionally, lack of time prevented discussion of all the questions included in the interview schedule.

3 The other principal components of the MS self-help regime were the taking of evening primrose oil, following a particular diet and exercise regime and ensuring adequate rest and relaxation.

REFERENCES

Baumann, B. (1961) 'Diversities in conceptions of health and physical fitness', *Journal Health and Human Behavior* 2: 39–46.

Blaxter, M. (1983) 'The causes of disease. Women talking', *Social Science and Medicine* 17: 59–69.

Blaxter, M. (1990) *Health and Lifestyles*, London: Routledge.

Blaxter, M. and Paterson, E. (1982) *Mothers and Daughters, A three generational study of health attitudes and behaviour*, London: Heinneman Educational Books.

Calnan, M. (1987) *Health and Illness, the Lay Perspective*, London: Tavistock Publications.

Cartwright, A. and Anderson, R. (1981) *General Practice Revisited, A second study of patients and their doctors*, London: Tavistock Publications.

Cornwell, J. (1984) *Hard Earned Lives – Accounts of health and illness from East London*, London: Tavistock Publications.

Crawford, M. (1984) 'A cultural account of "health": control, release, and the social body', in J.B. McKinlay (ed.) *Issues in the Political Economy of Health Care*, London: Tavistock Publications.

Davison, C., Davey-Smith, G. and Frankel, S. (1991) 'Lay epidemiology and the prevention paradox: the implications of coronary candidacy for health education', *Sociology of Health and Illness* 13: 1–19.

Freidson, E. (1970) *Profession of Medicine: A study of the sociology of applied medicine*, New York: Dodd Mead.

Hannay, D. (1979) *The Symptom Iceberg, A study in Community Health*, London: Routledge & Kegan Paul.

Herzlich, C. (1973) *Health and Illness, A social-psychological analysis*, London: Academic Press.

Locker, D. (1981) *Symptoms and Illness, the cognitive organisation of disorder*, London: Tavistock Publications.

Parsons, T. (1972) 'Definitions of health and illness in the light of American values and social structure', in E.G. Jaco (ed.) *Patients Physicians and Illness*, New York: Free Press.

Pill, R. and Stott, N.C. (1982) 'Concepts of illness causation and responsibility; some preliminary data from a sample of working class mothers', *Social Science and Medicine* 16: 43–52.

Pill, R. and Stott, N.C. (1985) 'Choice or Chance: further evidence on ideas of illness and responsibility for health', *Social Science and Medicine* 20: 981–91.

Pollock, K. (1984) 'Mind and Matter, A study of conceptions of health and illness among three groups of English families, with particular reference to Multiple Sclerosis, Schizophrenia and "Nervous Breakdown",' unpublished Ph.D. thesis, University of Cambridge.

Pollock, K. (1988) 'On the nature of social stress: production of a modern mythology', *Social Science and Medicine* 26: 381–92.

Sontag, S. (1979) *Illness as Metaphor*, London: Allen Lane.

Tuckett, D., Boulton, M., Olson, C. and Williams, A. (1985) *Meetings Between Experts, an approach to sharing ideas in medical consultations*, London: Tavistock Publications.

Twaddle, A. (1974) 'The concept of health status', *Social Science and Medicine* 8: 29–38.

Wadsworth, M.E.J. Butterfield, W.J.H. and Blaney, R. (1971) *Health and Sickness: the choice of treatment*, London: Tavistock Publications.

WHO (1973) *The International Pilot Study of Schizophrenia*, Geneva.

WHO (1975) *Schizophrenia: a multi-national study*, WHO Public Health Paper No. 63, Geneva.

WHO (1979) *Schizophrenia, an international follow-up study*, New York.

Williams, R. (1983) '*Concepts of health: an analysis of lay logic*', Sociology 17: 185–205.

Zborowski, M. (1952) 'Cultural components in responses to pain', *Journal of Social Issues* 8: 17–33.

Zola, I.K. (1973) 'Pathways to the doctor: from person to patient', *Social Science and Medicine* 7: 677–89.

4 Religion and illness

Rory Williams

There has long been a curious silence on the subject of religion in medical sociology, though it is beginning to be broken by new voices. It is not difficult to think of reasons for the silence. The rise of medical sociology in the 1960s occurred during a period of steep decline in churchgoing (Currie *et al.* 1977). The university culture during this period was antipathetic to religion (Wadsworth and Freeman 1983). Sociology in particular tended to treat religion as an epiphenomenon. The sociology of religion was dominated by the topic of secularization. And the sociology of illness took much of its agenda from medicine, and where it did not, was dominated by a monolithic picture of society in which overarching social conventions defined what is normal, and the ill were among many groups of deviants who struggled with, and variously renegotiated, accepted, evaded, or cheated these norms. If religion had a place in such a scheme, it was only detectable as the social cement in the conventional edifice, more of an obstruction than anything else to the spaces which people had made for themselves to live in. In short, medical sociology was itself highly secularized, even though many individual medical sociologists had some religious background and motivation, and it was developing on the liberal assumption that social life in its field of study had also become highly secularized.

The secularization of illness is itself a topic of great interest – diverse forms of this process have been discerned in the literature, and corresponding reverse processes have also been detected. But secularization and its reversals are by no means the only religious processes at work in the contemporary experience of illness. An equally striking tendency is the frequent divergence of institutional religion from personal systems of meaning, and systems of meaning are particularly important in the response to illness. But a major obstacle to a widespread consideration of these systems of meaning is the difficulty which many medical sociologists have in bringing into focus the idea of religion, as opposed to membership of an institutional church, and especially the idea of religion as something which, in its elementary forms, is very general and not necessarily supernatural.

Religion is not susceptible to a single definition, any more than health or illness is, and like health or illness its distinctive features shade off at varying points, in all its dimensions, into conceptions and practices which are universal. It is made up, amongst other things, of a scheme for interpreting the world, a moral vision which flows from that interpretation, a sense of individual and group identity, and a practice designed to symbolize and reaffirm all of these elements – all potential features of any culture or social movement.

Any study of symbolic practice, sense of identity, moral beliefs or schemes of interpretation is, therefore, in the antechamber of religion. Indeed it may already be dealing with religion unawares – for as an Aberdonian told me: 'This is religion – you very seldom talk about it'. At this level it is not particularly useful, other than for polemical purposes, to discriminate political and cultural movements from religions, for such movements begin to look like religions once they achieve, or once they become associated with movements which have achieved, sufficient generality of scope. If their scheme of interpretation attains cosmological dimensions, or their moral claims are universal; if their sense of identity is treated as constant for all future circumstances, and their symbols are treated as illuminating permanent truths about the world, they are beginning to crystallize into religious movements bearing a symbolic universe or sacred cosmos as their dynamic centre, which will be applied to interpret and bring coherence to new contexts and new events into the indefinite future (Luckmann 1967, Berger and Luckmann 1967). Here it is useful to distinguish between secularization and secularism: while secularization as we have it largely betokens an indifference to cosmic and moral universals, secularism argues consciously for its own moral universals within an atheist cosmology, and is up to this point itself a religion. Only beyond this point is it useful to distinguish religions which are secularist, or which remain this-worldly, and those which go further, seeking to transcend the natural world, like Theravada Buddhism, or to encounter God, like the religions of the Bible.

It follows from this way of looking at religion that it is simply the most enduring and dynamic form in which interpretive schemata, moral praxis, sense of identity and symbolic action are organically linked. That does not mean of course, that it is to be found, fully-fledged, in a large proportion of the contemporary Western autobiographies which come to the ear of a sociologist. It means that fragments of these elements are present in most autobiographies, organic connections of several elements in many, and the full crystallization in a minority. The dynamic nature of religion is not necessarily revealed in its ability fully to co-opt the majority at any one time, though this may have occurred in some periods, but in its capacity to reproduce itself in fresh contexts over long historical spans.

The initial task for the listening sociologist, therefore, is to learn to recognize religion in its dissolved as well as in its crystallized forms; and for this purpose the rest of this paper focuses especially on two broad categories of incomplete religious formation: institutional identity with little development of moral and interpretive schemata, and moral and interpretive development without institutional identity.

By institutional identity I mean a cluster of different but related things. At its strongest it would include avowed membership of a religious group or institution, appropriate religious practice, and a corresponding sense that 'we' and 'I' are people of such and such a kind, and as we should be. At its weakest it would typically be a mere assertion of institutional membership, without practice or moral identity ('I'm Church of England, but I'm not really religious'); or it would be a sense of a moral identity with no current membership or practice, and at best an acknowledgement of membership and instruction in the past ('I went to Sunday School and that, and I've always done my best to work hard and look after my family').

By moral and interpretive development I mean the formation of a generalized world view, whether simple or complex. Initially this may show itself only in the avowal of some universal moral imperative, often of a deceptively platitudinous kind. But there is often an interpretive back-up, which tacitly or explicitly hypothesizes the powers which control human life, and their limits, and thus denotes the scope of moral or religious behaviour. Some talk along these lines is reminiscent of the sociological theme of locus of control (Rotter 1966, Wallston et al. 1978), but it is far more complex than a division into internal versus external control. At the minimum, health talk counterposes the powers of the individual versus those of the society, and both versus the involuntary powers of the body and the natural world (Herzlich 1973); and in many cases it goes on to contrast both voluntary and mechanical powers with supernatural or psychic powers which, while not under human control, are responsive to human approach (Antonovsky 1979: 152–6). Thus moralities may be individualistic, political, fatalistic, or metaphysical in origin, or some combination of these, depending on the identification of the powers that control human life and the way they are seen to interact; and correspondingly illness may be God-given (a sacrifice, trial or punishment), a fate, a social role or a challenge to individual creativity (Williams 1990, Herzlich and Pierret 1984). Needless to say, such ideas may go with no religious identification of an institutional kind.

THE SOCIOGRAPHY OF RELIGION IN AND OUTSIDE INSTITUTIONAL FORMS

Before I outline the implications for health of these differing kinds of religious formation, it may be helpful to get a quantitative picture, however sketchy, of their frequency in a contemporary Western population. In particular, following the theme of this chapter, we need an impression of how often individual religion is formed on a predominantly institutional pattern, and how often on a predominantly moral and interpretive pattern, and in which traditions we may expect to find these developments.

The figures which follow are taken from two parallel surveys of random samples carried out during 1987 in Clydeside, one of 985 men and women aged around 35 from the general population (Macintyre *et al.* 1989), the other of 173 men and women aged 30–40 (mean 35) of South Asian descent in Glasgow, stratified to represent Muslims and non-Muslims in equal proportions, who were interviewed with pretranslated schedules in their first language (Ecob and Williams 1991). The established church in Scotland is the Church of Scotland, which is Presbyterian, but ethnic and religious minorities are prominent, especially Catholics (here mostly of Irish descent), and (to a much smaller extent) the religions practised in the north of the Indian subcontinent. Religious practice is commoner in Scotland, as in Wales and Ireland, than in England (Brierley 1982), but there has been a parallel decline in churchgoing (Currie *et al.* 1977), and Scotland shares most features of the secularization which has been seen in Britain generally.

The first stage of religious formation is however, in this population, almost universal. Nearly all these people, now in their thirties, had been given a religious identity at birth (98 per cent of the general population sample). It is the religious development of this population in adult life which has been most diverse. All these groups were asked whether they belonged to any religious group now, how often they went to services or religious activities, and how important religion was in their life. The question about importance was aimed at the dimension of moral and interpretive meaning, and a more specific question about religious ways of coping was added to see whether this sense of the importance of religion was extended into personal experience related to health. A list of 11 common ways of coping with stress (resting, taking exercise, etc.) was read out, one of which was religious activities or prayer, and respondents were asked to indicate how helpful they themselves found each of them. This question on the helpfulness of religion was closely correlated in Clydeside with the question on its importance, and 96 per cent of those who found religion quite or very helpful in this situation (98 per cent among South Asians) attributed some degree of importance to it. The question about importance does therefore seem to have elicited personal meanings.

These indications – current sense of religious identity and attendance on the one hand, and the importance attributed to religion on the other – can thus be used to draw a picture of differing levels of religious formation in the contemporary Clydeside population in early middle life (Table 4.1).

Table 4.1 Clydeside 35-year-olds, 1987: differing levels of religious formation

Level of religious formation	*N*	*%*
Currently belongs to no religious group, says religion not important, attends services less than once a month	233	23.8
Currently belongs to a religious group and/or says religion only a little bit important, attends services less than once a month	277	28.4
Attends services once a month or more, but says religion only a little or not important	65	6.6
Says religion quite or very important, but attends services less than once a month	113	11.5
Says religion quite or very important and attends services once a month or more	292	29.7
Total (MD = 5)	980	100.0

With the exception of principled secularists, who are generally found to be a very small proportion of British populations, it can be supposed that those who said religion was not important in their lives, and who did not usually attend services, represented the lowest level of religious formation (about a quarter of the population). Even at this level, people were still affected by the religious identity given them at birth, for nearly all (91 per cent) of them attended services occasionally, though for the most part only on special occasions such as funerals and marriages. In so far as these rites of passage centred on members of their familial and social circle who were born into the same church, a childhood identity was still occasionally accepted in deference to them, but it was not otherwise recognized as effective in the present.

The next level of religious formation is also relatively shallow – merely a retention of religious identity into adult life. This can be described as current subjective attachment (a sense of membership, or regarding religion as a little bit important) without either regular attendance (once a month or more) or serious personal meaning (religion quite or very important) – approximately another quarter of the population.

The remaining half of the Clydeside population, then, represent higher levels of religious formation; but from this point on the objective pathway of religious formation, through collective religious activity, and the subjective pathway, through the personal import of religion, often diverge, creating the institutional identity without development of personal meaning, or the development of meaning without institutional identity, to which I referred earlier. It is true that those who attended services regularly and who also thought religion was quite or very important were marginally in the majority; but over a quarter of those who thought religion quite or very important did not attend activities as often as once a month, and nearly a fifth of those who attended at that level thought religion was only a little bit important or not important in their own lives. Furthermore these overall figures mask considerable divergences between collective activity and personal meaning in the different religious groups, and it is now time to look at these.

Table 4.2 shows the extent to which people born into each religious group had retained that identity into middle life, attended collective religious activities, and felt their religion to be important in their own lives. Retention of identity was actually or virtually complete in the special sample of Muslims, Sikhs and Hindus. It was high among Catholics (79 per cent), and also in the small group who had no religious identity at birth. But retention was low amongst Protestants. The Church of Scotland had retained a little over half its self-identified members, and other Christian groupings only a small minority. On the whole defectors said they had no current institutional

Table 4.2 Clydeside 35-year-olds and Glasgow South Asians aged 30-40, 1987: retention of religious identity, attendance, and subjective importance of religion by religious group

Religious group at birth	*% with current religious group:*			*% attending once a month or more*	*% saying religion quite/very important in their life*	N
	same	*another*	*none*			
Church of Scotland	57	7	36	27	31	505
Anglican	23	29	48	18	25	44
Other Protestant (specified)	16	27	57	36	41	44
Protestant (unspecified)	18	26	56	18	31	39
Catholic	79	6	15	59	63	299
Muslim	100	0	0	38	99	90
Sikh	97	1	2	69	85	62
Hindu	90	10	0	34	85	18
None	83	17	83	11	22	18

membership, with the exception of those born into the smaller Protestant denominations.

The picture of collective activity is broadly consistent with this picture amongst Protestants, but it introduces new perspectives on the other groups. Collective activity was highest among those born into the Sikh and the Catholic faiths, and only moderate among those born into the Church of Scotland, the Hindu faith, and Islam (in this last case not so much among the men, 60 per cent of whom attended the mosque once a month or more, as among the women, most of whose practice is domestic). Collective activity was low among those born Protestant without further specification, and among those born into the Anglican communion, and not surprisingly it was lowest among those born with no religious identity.

Collective activity does not, however, determine personal meaning. The personal importance attributed to religion by those born into the different groups often follows a quite different pattern. Nearly all born Muslims, and the great majority of those born Sikh or Hindu, thought their religion quite or very important in their lives. So too did most born Catholics. Among the rest, two fifths of those born into the smaller Protestant denominations attached importance to religion, and around a quarter, more or less, of the remainder, including those born with no religious identity.

These results signal radical differences in the extent to which the personal meaning of the religions discussed here is centred in collective activity. Table 4.3 shows the proportion of those who felt religion was quite or very important in their lives, but who nevertheless did not attend collective activities regularly (at least once a month). Felt importance was seldom divorced from collective activity for born Catholics and born Sikhs; but over a third of serious Protestants did not attend collective activities regularly, and the majority of serious Muslims and Hindus did not do so (again with the qualification that among born Muslims, only 39 per cent of the serious male

Table 4.3 Clydeside 35-year-olds and Glasgow South Asians aged 30-40, 1987: subjective importance of religion by attendance

Religious group at birth	*% of those saying religion quite/very important who attend services <1 per month*	*% of those attending services 1+ per month who say religion only a little or not important*
Protestant/ Anglican	37	27
Catholic	17	11
Muslim	63	4
Sikh	27	8
Hindu	62	*

* N < 15

adherents did not attend regularly, while 81 per cent of serious female adherents did not do so).

Similarly there are also differences in the extent to which collective activity is part of an institutional identity with relatively little personal meaning. Among those attending public gatherings regularly, born Protestants were the likeliest to attach little or no personal importance to their religion. In other religious groups this was rare.

These differences in the balance between collective institutional activity and personal meaning occur in spite of the determined retention of religious identity and the intense importance attached to religion among Catholics and amongst those of South Asian descent. In both instances religion is the vital basis of moral identity for ethnic minorities which have faced adverse circumstances over a number of years. Yet Sikhs and Catholics on the one side, and Hindus and Muslim women on the other, demonstrate extremes in the collective and personal focus of religious life. This finding gives a new perspective to the similar and more familiar differences between Catholics and Protestants: for although institutional identity without personal meaning is obviously commoner among Protestants where the established church is Protestant, the important role played by individual or domestic systems of personal meaning among Protestants who ignore collective activities should not be underestimated in the light of similar patterns in other religions. In what follows, I turn to a discussion of Protestant institutional identities and Protestant systems of personal meaning in the context of illness, with a view to showing how these can be elicited by qualitative methods.

AUTOBIOGRAPHICAL MEANINGS OF RELIGION IN ILLNESS

The material that follows will illustrate these aspects of Protestantism from autobiographical interviews held with 70 Aberdonians aged 60 and over in 1979/80. The way in which they coped with illness, old age, the prospect of dying, and the experience of bereavement, and the influence on their thinking of the economic history of Aberdeen under capitalism, and its religious history under Protestantism, has been the subject of a full-scale monograph (Williams 1990). Here I use material from the fieldwork in a more brief and illustrative form, with particular attention to the ways in which incomplete levels of religious formation – incomplete, that is, in terms of an earlier Protestant tradition which stressed both the personal and the collective focus – can be recognized by the fieldworker who is interested both in health and illness and in systems of meaning.

Preserving life and preventing illness

The world of illness is bounded by normal health on the one hand and death on the other; some people never enter it, and some pass through it so rapidly that no question of controlling it arises. What arises instead is the preventive question of avoiding both illness and premature death.

The role of religion in this task of preservation hinges on a common equation, or perhaps more accurately a common coalescence, between the ideas of health and salvation, to both of which virtuous living can be expected, depending on circumstances, to conduce. Although the ascetic and dietary practices of religions often differ strikingly, as do the good works to which adherents are directed, elements of them may well lead to material as well as spiritual betterment, whether by accident or design.

At first, and in relation to illness without any particular mortal threat, there may be a deceptive pragmatism about recipes for prevention in the Western world. People will assent with varying degrees of enthusiasm to the idea that exercise, a sensible diet, no smoking and moderate drinking are the requisites for health, and it may be supposed that they owe these convictions to medical advice and education. It is only with more extended listening that one notices certain things which are puzzling. Aberdonians, for example, who heartily endorse the idea of keeping active, may respond to the doctor's advice to do exercises by muttering 'Awa' wi' ye'. Worse still, when told by the doctor to rest instead, they may suddenly kick over the traces without ceremony:

> 'The GP spoke to me, but I said I'd rather die feeling the way I do now than live the way I was before.'

Clearly something else is happening here than a docile internalization of medical science. And when a more principled reason is given for such an attitude, its scope is often broad and includes a self-characterization of a strong, declaratory sort:

> 'Are there things you do to keep healthy?'
> 'No – just, I'm never off my feet. I'm always going about doing work and helping somebody else.'

Such claims to identity may of course reflect a lifetime of successful management of diseases remediable by physical exercise and social involvement – say circulatory problems combined with a tendency to depression; but they also look suspiciously like moral claims, an impression which is strengthened by any prolonged exposure to Aberdonian attitudes to work.

In the instances so far quoted morality is only implicit – the text could still be read as a set of nostrums for health, even if idiosyncratic and intolerant of advice; at other times, though, morals poke through unmistakably. The way in which even medically correct attitudes are phrased may give the game away:

> 'I told them I don't drink and I don't smoke and I don't go to bingo and I don't go with the mannies [men].'

Even without the bingo, which the most unobservant eye would notice is not prominent in health education manuals, there is a certain non-medical resonance about this list which may prompt enquiry, and elicit the Salvation Army childhood which lies behind it. In other cases, one falls over the hidden moral or religious assumption by sheer accident:

> 'And when did you first become conscious of the importance of food for health?'
> 'Eh, to tell you the truth, I think I have inherited that from my mother, and, I think, her grandmother – her mother and grandmother before her, as I'm led to believe, were the salt of the earth. They knew what was good for them, and they were healthy, and they valued their health and were willing to give up everything, you know, for to be well. Which in my book is everything, because if you are occupying a hospital bed you are costing the health service a lot of money.'
> 'Yes, Yes. And eh, were they Aberdeen people, your ... eh?'
> 'No. My grandmother was fisher. They came from Fife, Fifeshire.'
> 'Fifeshire, yes.'
> 'But they were the good old religious kin' o' people, you know.'
> 'Yes. Yes.'
> 'God-fearing, that's the word. God-fearing, but eh, as my grandmother used to say, look after the pot and other things'll look after themselves.'

If one is to account for all these phenomena (and of course the examples given are purely illustrative) it is hard to avoid the conclusion that, whether at a more or less consciously moralizing level, a health-giving value is being asserted not for particular elements like exercise in the abstract, and not only for remedies scientifically proven to help particular conditions, as exercise helps locomotor conditions and rest helps angina, but for a whole way of life in which working and eating, welldoing and abstinence, are combined in a virtuous balance and handed down from one generation to another.

Whether this way of life gives not only health but salvation is then a matter for careful exploration; and one circumstance in which such assumptions may be revealed is in accounting for a death which breaches them.

The sudden or premature death of an adult occasions special grief in most cultures, but the cultural resources for making sense of the event differ. A soldier's, a martyr's, a consumptive's, an accident victim's death have been given different meanings in different periods. In Western culture, though, according to one argument (Parsons *et al.* 1972), the most prominent tendency is to see such events as adventitious and senseless; for the Judaeo-Christian tradition defines each life as a gift from God, to be given back to God only when it has fulfilled its natural span. There is some truth in this for the Jewish tradition, and for those Protestant traditions which give weight to a literal and unselective reading of the Old Testament; for the fifth commandment ('Honour thy father and thy mother, that thy days may be long upon the land which the Lord thy God giveth thee') is amongst a number of references which can be heard to offer long life to the virtuous.[1] But in most of the Christian tradition, the New Testament provides a powerful counterbalance, as well as a prism for reinterpreting the Old Testament, emphasizing the reversals of the Beatitudes and the often-repeated paradox that those who lose their lives shall save them. And at the individual level the facts of pre-industrial life expectancy will often have fitted better with the New rather than the Old Testament emphasis.

For these reasons it is not surprising to find that in listening to accounts of such deaths there are at least two different senses which can be made of them. The first is perhaps the most easily overlooked, for it does not issue in a contradiction, and therefore gives rise to few extended passages of discussion and little agonizing. Indeed reference to it in the context of premature death may slip by only in an isolated proverbial allusion, inviting rapport and eluding the need for questioning:

> 'You canna go before your time.'
>
> 'When your time's up, it's up. I'm a great believer in that.'
>
> 'If it's God's will she has to go, well, she'll go whenever she's ready.'

These were not fatalistic statements in the usual sense of that word. In Aberdeen, interestingly, most of them occurred in the context of vigorous efforts to acquire information, reach rational decisions, and exercise the maximum possible control over the course of illness or threats to life, and none was used to justify inaction. Rather they related to the idea that age, statistical expectations, and what might seem the natural time to die for humans collectively, were irrelevant to what was essentially an individual destiny, in which readiness was achieved at a particular point in a personal story. In the various stories I was told, this point could be one of hopes fulfilled, or of tragedy and division resolved. Marriage, the birth of children, success at work could all provide auspicious turning points when death entered, not indeed as a welcome visitor, but without shattering the meaning of life. And in lives already made incoherent by family quarrels or personal wrongs, a movement of reconciliation restored coherence and rendered death ultimately intelligible.

There was a clear contrast, however, between this attitude to premature deaths and one based on the justice of a natural term of life. There was no difference in the two kinds of account in the age of death or the length of time since the death, but ideas of a natural term occasioned especially bitter and long-lived grief, and the story was frequently accompanied by tears. Further, the way in which the contradiction was expressed was unambiguously a matter of religion, and found similar form in the words of widely differing characters:

> 'She always went to the church and the Guild, and so did I, and it makes you think why did it happen to her?'

> 'She went to church. I used to say, "Oh don't speak to me about church." And then she died so young.'

> 'She was quite enthusiastic about going to church, which we did a lot, and she was keen, just as her mother was, and the routine was we rushed off to hymns. After she went, I felt a bit ... bitter, I must admit, selfishly so perhaps – because she was a very good type of woman, was very popular, was just ... very good.'

> 'He came home from church, and he felt, well, everything's going to be all right, and this sermon was to him. And she died the next day. And he just thought, you know ... his faith sort of left him.'

Now the other thing which clearly characterized this experience was what I have called institutional identity without a developed world view. This is already apparent in some of the quotations just given, where two of the speakers intimate that they were not themselves as deeply involved in church life as the person who died. And indeed, while contributing and, if able, attending, they were all otherwise remarkable for silence or scepticism on matters of cosmology or morality. Their relation to the church was rather a form of contract between the membership and the minister. In the Church of Scotland (the principal church involved here) the minister, always a graduate, and the church itself, should ideally be fully paid for by the local congregation. And in return (according to the contractual view) the minister looks after the welfare of the congregation, calling in particular on the sick and the bereaved. It was this godly commonwealth, then, if one may put it so, comprising minister and paid-up attenders, that was felt to have a claim on the promise for each individual of a full term of life.

Among those whose religion has formed only as an institutional identity, then, one may look, at any rate in Scotland, for a characteristic conception of the way illness is prevented and life preserved, one which elides the ideas of health and salvation. It accepts a way of life handed down, chiefly identified (for its proponents are chary of personal moralizing) with hard work and good food, which is effective in preventing illness and promoting resistance to it; and which, when accompanied by a due reciprocity between the minister and the membership of the local church, is virtuous in the eyes of God, and has a claim on divine promises of a natural term of life. But much even of these assumptions remains tacit, and emerges only under the pressure of experiences which contradict them.

Curing illness

When curable illness strikes, the concerns that people have are not only to do with evaluating their symptoms, deciding whether to consult the doctor and others, and carrying out the regimen their advisers recommend; they are also to do with the reasons why they should have lost their resistance to illness in the first place. And so along with the processes of lay diagnosis, medical consultation and treatment, there is often a moral discourse going on which reinvokes the same powers as are felt to contribute to preventing illness and preserving life.

With those who are institutionally identified with religion and nothing more, or indeed with those whose sense of identity lies only in possession of the qualities approved in their culture, this means a reassertion of the same healing powers of hard work and good eating, and, for some, church membership. But those who have developed moral or metaphysical ideas tend to add to this repertoire.

Moralists, as I have said, add benevolence and abstinence to their list of healthy behaviours, and they may draw on various sources to reinforce their argument. In Scotland, those who reject supernatural religion tend to appeal to socialist thought, as is not surprising in a Labour stronghold, though apostles of competition can also be found who use Adam Smith and sociobiology to similar effect. Scottish socialism is not necessarily opposed to Christianity, though it may be construed so; on the contrary it is usually felt to elaborate and specify at a collective level what Christianity stands for at an individual level, and it is not hard to see why this should lead to the twin imperatives of altruism and self-denial. Competition, on the other hand, can be felt, in line with the ideology of fee-paying schools in the past, to develop both physical and mental functions – *mens sana in corpore sano* – and so promotes health through a balanced life; abstinence is again reinforced by the need to train these functions, and even altruism may be endorsed to some extent by a theory of competition between groups. This group psychology may also be used to explain religion, even to legitimate it, though this is clearly a very Durkheimian religion not far removed from school spirit.

All this of course broadly reflects the late nineteenth- and twentieth-century debates of Evangelicalism and Presbyterianism with socialism and *laissez-faire* liberalism (Brown 1987); but in the health context metaphysical beliefs do not express themselves through moral and political principles alone. They may also invoke additional powers of prayer and supernatural grace, and stories of miracles may be heard which claim that something has occurred, not which breaches natural law, but which answers prayer or faith at a time when it seems less than likely, and proves to be a biographical turning point:

> 'He told me the flesh might be all grown through the plate, and the plate might be corroded, and he mightn't be able to get it out; and also the wound might get infected. ... But I have a great faith, as you know, and it's helped greatly in my life, and I said I would try. I had three blood transfusions during the operation, but he got the plate out, and a few days later Mr Burnett came and sat by the bed and put his hand on mine, and said, "Do you believe in miracles?" And I said, "Yes, I do, I do believe, because miracles do happen". And he said, "Well, it's a miracle".'

Such events are not just a matter of individual faith; they are also communal achievements, attributed as much to the prayers of others – friends, family, church fellowships – as to those of the person concerned; and of course they are also, and primarily, divine interventions as well, thus representing a harmonious synergy of God, the individual and the collective.

Curing powers, therefore, like preventive powers, are understood within a limited number of interpretive schemes. Power may reside in the social order and an inherited way of life seen as a natural, beneficial and unalterable phenomenon; or in the same phenomenon seen as the creation of a provident and just God. Such interpretations are often only half conscious and vulnerable to disaster. Alternatively power may reside in a moral theory of collective action, or in a moral theory of individual responsibility, either of which may be seen as consonant with religious revelation, and either of which may be used to supplant it. Such interpretations are highly conscious, and can deal positively with disaster, though they may bear a heavy weight of self-blame in failure. Finally power may reside in a complex co-operation between God and the faith of both individual and collective. This kind of interpretation is conscious but often secretive or inarticulate. However the strength of all these interpretive schemata depends on one further situation with which they all have occasionally to cope.

When cure fails

The persistence of illness and disability poses an inescapable threat to all the interpretive schemes so far discussed. That is perhaps obvious for those that see the social order as both unalterable and benevolent. Chronic illness then places them in a situation at best of exile from the social order, and at worst of punishment: exile if the controlling powers are blind and mechanical, in which case the individual experience, so contrary to the general process of society, may be explained by chance or fate; punishment if the controlling power is an overmastering God, in which case there may be a search for voluntary or involuntary misdoings. In either case the implications are entirely negative.

For moralists, whether individualist or collectivist in their bent, the possibilities are more complex. Chronic illness may be the consequence of voluntary misdoing, but by the same token the context may allow the opportunity for correction. For individualists that may be hopeful, but on the other hand persisting illness which is read as a failure to correct then brings double damnation. For collectivists the situation is easier but less optimistic: the persistence of individual chronic illness cannot refute their belief that collective control is possible and desirable, but even if it is achieved it need not be universally efficacious, and the chances of individual improvement are equally compromised.

Even for the power of prayer, understood without elaboration or qualification, chronic illness is a threat. Absolute proponents of prayer may then be tempted to depreciate the faith of the sufferer, or of themselves – and this is perhaps the most threatening consequence of all.

In all these instances chronic illness poses a question which needs a creative resolution. In a fully-developed religious world view this necessity is a recognized topic – the problem of suffering, of theodicy (Weber 1947), the 'justification of God'; but for religion which is less fully formed, limited to a fixed morality or sense of identity, the need for creativity may be unperceived, though it is no less present.

In Aberdeen the difficulty centred most painfully around the health-giving properties of normal work and activity. It followed from this conception that incapacity negated both normal identity and the power of recovery. In this situation people were 'lost', no longer themselves, 'socially dead', 'finished', 'done', 'a poor thing'. The powerful Aberdonian work ethic, associated with the moral value of helping others and benefiting the community, and bringing with it the reward, or for some the blessing, of health, had this formidable obverse side; and it was overwhelmingly the case that the kind of religion which was formed only on an institutional identity, or only on a social or individual morality, was unable, in chronic illness, to break free from this sense of a loss of self.

In Aberdeen, a creative resolution of this difficulty was in fact only possible in any systematic way through an elaborated world view in which morality was supported and qualified by a metaphysical or mystical belief. While this was typically reinforced by church practice, it could also be sufficient by itself. Sheila Hannay was no churchgoer, and she made gentle satire of acquaintances who were too 'Christian'. She had read D.H. Lawrence in her youth, and he still seemed to her to be a touchstone. But her mockery of Presbyterian orthodoxy would have been entirely deceptive if it had been taken as a rejection of religion; for late in our talk a number of implicit nuances became explicit:

> 'I believe in God, you see – well when I say God, I think there is something, and I find that I can reach him if I'm in the country or even walking through the little park there, looking at the trees, and I think "That's God". I mean it's what it's all about, isn't it? It's all round you, it's in you, and it's for life. And I think there's an element of – I get a little strength from prayer; I think I believe in prayer, and that's truly as far as I would go.'

This suddenly made sense of earlier discussions when she had been talking of her experience of a serious crisis in her illness:

> 'You see, if you've had a really bad illness you realize what life is all about, the values of life. You've got to get your values sorted out and how trivial all this [owning possessions] is. This is all just escape. It's all rubbish really. The real things in life are having good friends, and health, and love if you can get it.'
>
> 'Is this something, when you had your illness ...?'
>
> 'Oh, I've felt like that for a long time. Yes, I would think every time you had a bad illness you .... the first thing you do is you go down the street and you think, "The flowers in the garden are wonderful", you know, and you look at the sky and the trees and you think: "Oh God, it's good to be alive". And to keep remembering that, I think, is important.'

There is a precise link here, in the trees in the 'little park there' of the first quotation which was down at the end of her street, and the flowers and the sky and the trees in the garden of the second quotation, which also are seen 'down the street': evidently both references are to the same place and typical experience. Thus the real things of life identified in the course of her disabling and occasionally life-threatening illness – the 'good friends, and health, and love if you can get it', which contrast with the triviality, escape and 'rubbish' of possessions – were found by an experience in the garden at the end of her street, or in the country, of something that is 'all round you' and 'in you', that is 'what it's all about' and is 'for life'. And evidently that something was hard to name with the big word 'God', which echoed with difficult associations, and once sounded had to be quickly silenced: 'Well, when I say God ...'. But it was nevertheless the only word which would do, and could be heard in its true timbre if taken by surprise: 'That's God', or 'Oh God, it's good to be alive'. And in this way she entered into a state which she recognized with similar hesitancy as prayer, from which, whatever it was, she got 'a little strength'.

Now the importance of this experience for her illness was in the fact that it had enabled her to 'sort out' her values and decide which were 'of life' and which were 'just escape'. Owning possessions, as the second quotation shows, was just escape; but equally downplayed was the Aberdonian ethic of work and being useful:

> 'They can't live unless they're doing something for somebody. Now I think that must be terrible. I don't think there's anything wrong in being selfish, like I am a bit, and being good to yourself. ... Well, they have a reason for living – that's their reason for living. I don't have to have a reason for living, the reason I'm alive is that my father and my mother made me, brought me forth, and I don't have to justify the fact that I'm alive.'

This did not mean that she rejected the health-giving value of effort and activity; but she refused to invest it with ultimate moral authority, and instead spoke of it as a means to an end, or as something she enjoyed in itself:

> 'I go for my walk in the morning because I've plenty of energy in the morning. And I walk and walk and walk until I'm dead tired, you know; I really like to extend myself because I think that's the only way I'm going to keep myself fit. I can't jog, so I do the other thing, and I'm keen on that because when I was younger I used to play golf a lot and I liked riding, but I can't do these things now, you see, so that's how I try and keep fit.'

This qualified, conditional view of activity subjected it to her own needs, for health, or simply for what she 'liked' and was 'keen on'; and this enabled her to see nothing wrong in being 'good to yourself'. Her sense of identity, her 'reason for living', which lay in her experience simply of being alive and in what was 'for life', remained unimpaired by being ill, incapacitated, and unable to work or do housework, or be useful to others, and as a result, she had developed a creative response to her illness which allowed her to seize on whatever alternatives were available:

> 'Well, I learned to give up things, that was the first lesson, I suppose I

> learned to enjoy things when they were available to be enjoyed. I've always snatched at pleasure when it was available ... I've always snatched the moment and I've never regretted it, even if I've made horrible mistakes. I don't regret them, it's all part of living.'

Here we see, then, that a capacity to deal flexibly with illness, to give up without regrets when incapacity makes that unavoidable, and to grasp alternatives as they arise, has become a valid identity in itself: 'I've always snatched the moment'. And that identity is not lost with incapacity, and with the failure to meet the health-giving normality of work and activity, because it is sustained by a mystical world view which, while entirely individualistic, is in some ways a quite highly developed form of religion, with a self-reinforcing practice of prayer and a capacity to endorse and reproduce a continuing sense of identity and an adaptive response in difficult circumstances. Thus the knot which the defeat of health poses to any interpretive scheme of health-giving powers, including religious schemes, can itself be untied by religion – not indeed one formed only on institutional identity, but one which adds to that the development of both moral and metaphysical interpretation, or even which relies solely on such interpretation in a form of mystical individualism.

CONCLUSION

I have argued that religion has been neglected in medical sociology, for a range of historical reasons, one of which has been the unconsidered identification of religion, in a subdiscipline largely formed on secular liberal assumptions, with churchgoing. The more pervasive and multidimensional picture of it which I have drawn here is one more familiar to sociologists of religion than of health. And it may be that some would still wish to argue that the subject matter of this paper is not so much religion as something else, under which religion can be subsumed.

Perhaps the standard candidate for an alternative description of my subject matter is ideology. This term has the satisfactory property of seeming to include any collection of ideas, from general concepts to self-images, while at the same time suggesting that a powerful sociological theory of ideology is at hand which will enable us to ask the necessary questions about them. But there is an important flaw in this comfortable association which is often overlooked. It is that the theory concerned asks a highly specific and limited set of questions about ideology as it defines it, which by no means covers all ideas in any context, much less all the questions one would wish to ask about ideas in general. In a scrupulous and wide-ranging recent survey of the subject, John Thompson defines the theoretical topic of ideology as 'the ways in which meaning serves to establish and sustain relations of domination'

(Thompson 1990). This is a question of great interest to medical as to other sociologists, but there are other questions of equal, even of prior, importance. One of the most interesting is in a sense the opposite of the monolithic Durkheimian question of domination: it concerns the ways in which meaning enables, making it possible for individuals to act, to share, and to enter into a fruitful relationship with the world both within and beyond the social order. Undoubtedly such meanings can at times be adapted to dominate us; but medical sociologists should be the first to recognize that one of the primary uses of words is to heal or, failing that, to transcend, suffering.

A second candidate for an alternative name for my subject matter in this paper is culture. But culture is too vast a term in one way, too narrow in another. Even if we adopt a more specific Geertzian conception of culture which focuses on symbolic forms, beliefs and values, the majority of these in any culture are at a low level of generality, and are seen as context-bound. Religion is only a part of culture in this sense, being an attempt, whether by individuals or by groups, to find a permanent identity, or to discern what is of permanent truth and value in the culture, and to reorient practice towards these things, while at the same time it usually introduces further symbols of other identities, or of things seen to be of permanent truth and value in other cultures and other times. It transcends the local, synchronic character of culture, and so as well as growing out of what is local and present it acts as a disturbing, re-orienting influence which interrogates what is local and present against what is and has been elsewhere and at other times. And for this reason it has an exceptionally long-lasting power of reproducing itself, far outstripping political and economic systems, which in itself should be of interest to sociology.

Thus while studies of ideology and culture must always be of interest to sociologists, they are an insufficient framework in which to ask the sorts of questions posed here. For these questions a concept of religion – or of some equivalent which encompasses the attempt to formulate permanent truths and values and to read these back into practice – is necessary.

With such a concept of religion (or its equivalent) a number of questions could be asked by medical sociologists in particular. The first set are questions of comparative history and anthropology: how far, and in what ways, are people in the contemporary West indifferent to issues of identity, morality or cosmology in facing health and illness, compared with other places and other times? Are they more indifferent (as theorists of secularization would argue), and if so, is this a new and singular phenomenon, derived from forces of rationalization in developing capitalism and bureaucracy (Wilson 1982), or is it merely one phase in a spectrum of cultural possibilities which have all manifested themselves in the preindustrial world (Douglas

1973)? Or do people in the West merely form their religion in a different, more individualistic way (Luckmann 1967)?

Second there are questions of comparative religion which are of particular importance for mutual understanding in a multicultural society. What do different religious traditions (including secularist traditions) offer, or fail to offer, in dealing with health and illness? How do they shape the explanations sought, the behaviour which prevents or cures, the adaptation to what is incurable, and the passage through death and bereavement? Doctors, nurses and patients have to understand one another over these things, as do all who seek to cope creatively or to comfort and support.

Third there are questions about the relations between religion (including secularist traditions) and medicine (or its alternatives). How far is contemporary medical explanation compatible with, or exclusive of, different patterns of religious explanation? What points of harmony or tension exist between medical practice and different religious values? How far have the points of tension led to alternative medicine, or alternative religions?

Finally there are questions of great interest about religion as both a product of social experience and a creator of social experience. To see it as exclusively one or the other leads to paradoxical results: a religion which does not respond to the life experience of a particular place and time can scarcely be an influence on it, while one which is entirely the product of a place and time can scarcely reproduce itself. Religion is a dialogue between a tradition and a form of life, but the particular shape which is taken by the dialogue is often important. Changes in life experience may lead people to select a different balance of emphases in the tradition, or may add to the tradition, or may be felt to make some parts of the tradition irrelevant; on the other hand tensions in the tradition, or charismatic upsurges, may cause divisions, or generate resolutions, which in turn leave a longstanding mark on life experience. In Aberdeen, I have argued, a longstanding mark of this kind was left by the debates of the Reformation (Williams 1990).

In all these questions, qualitative work and ethnographic listening of a careful, empathetic and deeply interesting kind can add a much fuller dimension to the quantitative, institutional and historical data which currently form most of the background. It is partly because worlds are not only socially but also religiously constructed that worlds of illness differ so greatly.

ACKNOWLEDGEMENTS

I am very grateful to my colleague Kate Hunt, who made available the data on Protestant and Catholic affiliation in Clydeside which is analysed in the second section of this paper. She and Kenneth Mullen have also made helpful comments on the text.

NOTE

1 See e.g. Exodus 20.12, 23.25f.; Leviticus 26; Dueteronomy. 7.12f., 28; Psalms 1, 34.12f., 37.

REFERENCES

Antonovsky, A. (1979) *Health, stress and coping*, San Francisco: Jossey-Bass.

Berger, P.L. and Luckmann, T. (1967) *The social construction of reality*, London: Allen Lane.

Brierley, P. (ed.) (1982) *The UK Christian Handbook: 1983 Edition*, London: The Evangelical Alliance, The Bible Society and MARC Europe.

Brown, C.G. (1987) *The social history of religion in Scotland since 1730*, London: Methuen.

Currie, R., Gilbert A. and Horsley, L. (1977) *Churches and churchgoers: patterns of church growth in the British Isles since 1700*, Oxford: Oxford University Press.

Douglas, M. (1973) *Natural Symbols*, Harmondsworth: Penguin.

Ecob, R. and Williams, R. (1991) 'Sampling Asian minorities to assess health and welfare', *J. Epidemiol. Comm. Health* 45: 93–101.

Herzlich, C. (1973) *Health and illness: a social psychological analysis*, tr. H.D. Graham, London: Academic Press.

Herzlich, C. and Pierret J. (1984) *Malades d'hier, malades d'aujourd'hui*, Paris: Payot.

Luckmann, T. (1967) *The invisible religion*, London: Macmillan.

Macintyre, S., Annandale, E., Ecob, R., Ford, G., Hunt, K., Jamieson, B., MacIver, S., West, P. and Wyke, S. (1989) 'The West of Scotland Twenty–07 Study: health in the community', in Martin, C. and McQueen, D. (eds), *Readings for a new public health*, Edinburgh: Edinburgh University Press.

Parsons, T., Fox, R.C. and Lidz V.M. (1972) 'The "gift of life", and its reciprocation', *Social Research* 39: 367–415.

Rotter, J.B. (1966) 'Generalised expectancies for internal versus external control of reinforcement', *Psychological Monographs* 80, no. 1.

Thompson, J.B. (1990) *Ideology and modern culture: critical social theory in the era of mass communication*, London: Polity Press.

Wadsworth, M.E.J. and Freeman, S.R. (1983) 'Generation differences in beliefs: a cohort study of stability and change in religious beliefs', *British Journal of Sociology* 34: 416–37.

Wallston, K.A., Wallston, B.S. and DeVellis, R. (1978) 'Development of the Multidimensional Health Locus of Control (MHLC) scales', *Health Education Monographs* 6, no. 2.

Weber, M. (1947) 'The social psychology of the world religions', in Gerth, H.H. and Mills C.W., *From Max Weber*, London: Kegan Paul.

Williams, R. (1990) *A Protestant legacy: attitudes to death and illness among older Aberdonians*, Oxford: Oxford University Press.

Wilson, B. (1982) *Religion in sociological perspective*, Oxford: Oxford University Press.

5 Chronic illness and the pursuit of virtue in everyday life

Gareth Williams

This chapter examines some of the ways in which society is represented by individuals through discussions of the impact of chronic illness and disablement upon them. Using an approach that is nowadays referred to as narrative analysis, I focus in detail on one individual as a case within whose account the workings of various societal forces can be discerned. The themes arising out of this are then given more general interpretation. I argue that in articulating the experience of illness in relation to their social milieux individuals elaborate moral discourses based on their own biographical experiences which often stand counter to the dominant rhetoric of both professionals and politicians.

INTRODUCTION

> The real moral objection is to relaxation in the security of possession, the enjoyment of wealth with the consequence of idleness and the temptations of the flesh, above all of distraction from the pursuit of a righteous life.
>
> (Weber 1976: 157)

It could be argued that health, like wealth, is neither good nor bad in itself. What is good is the self-disciplined activity which, according to Protestantism and Mrs Thatcher, produces them; and their absence is a sure sign of gluttony and sloth. Representations of health as a virtue, as a matter of right conduct, and illness as a sign of sinfulness and a warning to the individual to alter his or her behaviour, have deep roots in our Puritan traditions (Wear 1985). Illness may not itself be regarded as a sin, but the beliefs and behaviours which are claimed to give rise to illness are increasingly portrayed in terms of human wickedness by many of those engaged in the mission of promoting the nation's health (Rodmell and Watt 1986). This perspective on health may be seen as one expression of an individualistic ideology which leads to the blaming of individuals for the misfortunes they suffer, while preventing them from perceiving the relationships between the traps of their private lives and the structures of power and privilege in society (Mills 1970).

Individualism, ethical and methodological, represents a powerful current running through the political and economic life of Western society (Lukes 1973), and a tough strand of voluntarism has characterized the fabric of British social services since their inception – not surprisingly, in view of the virtual non-existence of such services up until 1900 (Parker and Mirrlees 1988). Both individualism as an ideology and voluntarism as an approach to welfare have enjoyed something of a resurgence during the 1980s. The sight of students, for example, standing on campus collecting money for one or other group of 'deserving poor' has become increasingly familiar and almost natural. At the same time questions have been voiced about the capacity of the post-war collectivist, tax-based welfare system to cope with the rapid increase in 'dependency groups' in Western societies (Illsley 1981). However, attitudes to the provision of welfare are riddled with ambiguity. Although formal surveys of opinion show that British people still support the principle of meeting a range of social needs through state intervention (West *et al.* 1984; Taylor-Gooby 1987), it is equally clear that individuals find abhorrent the idea of themselves and their families as being 'dependent' (Locker 1983); and the ideologists of the New Right have tugged insistently at this ontological uneasiness.

In trying to understand the ideological drifts that have contributed to an apparent loss of faith in the welfare state along with a renewal of interest in various manifestations of voluntarism we should recognize that: 'To be an individual has historic connotations of self-reliance, confidence, self-affirmation' (Sennett and Cobb 1973: 66). These connotations ripple through human experience in such a way that the ideology has its most powerful effects not on opinions expressed in answer to direct questions from professional strangers, but in the deeper recesses of social psychology which inform the practices of everyday life (Billig 1982). It is at this level that the tendency to blame the victim for those phenomena such as cancer and crime, which indicate both personal troubles and public issues, finds fertile soil.

The aim of this chapter is to examine daily life with chronic illness in order to elucidate the ways in which categorical notions, particularly about dependence and independence, interact with the situated pragmatism of everyday life (Heller 1984; Wright 1985; Anderson and Bury, 1988).

Using material from in-depth interviews with people with rheumatoid arthritis (RA), I will look at the characteristic ways in which society is represented through individuals' discussions of the impact of chronic illness and disablement upon them. The interpretation is undertaken through the detailed exegesis of an illustrative case followed by discussion of the general themes arising from it. I conclude by considering the wider implications of my analysis for the way in which we think about disablement.

DATA AND METHODS

The data employed in this paper were collected through the medium of semi-structured interviews with twenty-nine people suffering from RA of at least five years' duration. The people were interviewed at the start of the 1980s when 'Thatcherism', in the more or less clear sense in which we have come to understand it since its departure (Hall 1988; Skidelsky 1988), was an uncertain silhouette. The respondents were contacted through the out-patients' departments of two teaching hospitals in a large British city and were subsequently interviewed in their own homes. It cannot be claimed that these people are representative of RA sufferers in general – they have had many years of illness and disability and prolonged experience of treatment. For the purposes of an investigation of this sort, however, the nature of the generalization in which I am interested involves turning the issue around and asking: what is representative, characteristic or typical of the society in question in its impact on the people interviewed (Sennett and Cobb 1973). The interviews yielded lengthy accounts which move in and out of a variety of subjects of concern: some directly related to arthritis, others not. Topics for the interviews had been decided upon in advance but other significant themes emerged from analysis of the data and were incorporated as the study progressed. All the interviews were recorded on tape and then transcribed for detailed analysis.

Data produced in interviews such as these can be given different readings depending on the aims of the analysis and the epistemological assumptions which are brought to it. As Gouldner has argued: 'Domain assumptions about man and society are built not only into substantive social theory but into methodology itself' (Gouldner 1971: 49). For this reason, personal accounts can be used, on the one hand, as factual reports on daily life which provide usable information for practitioners and professionals about social problems arising out of the experience of disability (Locker 1983; Anderson and Bury 1988). On the other hand, they may be seen as complex expressions of subjective experience (Conrad 1987), forming narrative reconstructions or re-enactments (Williams 1989; Gilsenan 1989) which can be understood only against the wider background of person and society. While the former approach assumes the relationship between language and social reality to be 'designative' and aims primarily to report, the latter presupposes a recognition of the relationship as being also 'expressive' and seeks to interpret and understand (Runciman 1983; Taylor 1985). In this paper I approach the words of my interviewees as responses to my questions about their arthritis which give voice to powerful and complex values and beliefs which form the accompaniments of their chronic illness (Corbin and Strauss, 1987).

THE MORAL ACCOMPANIMENTS OF CHRONIC ILLNESS IN AN INDIVIDUAL LIFE

Mrs Fields (this is not her real name) was a sixty-two-year-old woman who had had RA for approximately eight years. Her husband had died of cancer about two years prior to our meeting and she now lived alone, but in close proximity to relatives and friends. The town in which she lives had once been a centre of the cotton industry – an industry in which she had been employed for some years – but like many towns and cities in north-west England this one had seen better times. Before visiting her at home I had seen her in consultation with the rheumatologist at a teaching hospital in the city a few miles from her home. My impression was of a 'good patient': she was polite, deferential, and did not ask too many awkward questions. Over the years her arthritis had been treated with a variety of powerful anti-rheumatic drugs, such as gold injections and steroids which, she informed me with a touch of pride, she had 'accepted ... with no side-effects'. At the time I met her the physician was especially pleased because she had become a willing if rather nervous participant in the clinical trial of a new drug.

Doctor knows best

Her attitude to the doctors' dealings with her body was characterized by trust; relinquishing control over her body for the purposes of treatment was a necessary prerequisite to what she called 'independence' – a general social state the value of which clearly outweighed the cost in terms of periodic entry into the sick role:

> 'My thoughts are now that I've got nothing to worry about as regards treatment. Dr Jones's team is there to give it to me. I can just lock up here and go down there, and then come back here and become independent again.'

Abandonment of responsibility for her body as the receptacle of disease did not imply a passive stance towards its disabling consequences, or that she was 'giving up' on her life as a whole. Indeed, she concentrated on controlling just those things which she perceived as being within her power. Responding to a question about her daily activities before and after the onset of arthritis, she said: 'I do more ... yes, I do more, because the more you sit under it, the more you're apt to make it seize-up, which is no good'.

From Mrs Fields's point of view, therefore, a clear line could be drawn between the progression of her disease as being something over which she had little or no direct control, and the severity of the disabling symptoms of the disease, against which she felt compelled to assume a posture of resistance. Moreover, she fully understood that the disadvantages she experienced in relation to her daily life emerged from the interaction between herself and the environment. The seeming intractability of the environment sometimes produced a sense of panic which she struggled to overcome by looking at hazards pragmatically: 'If you find it hard when you first start doing something, leave it and go back another day, then it just clicks'.

The social basis of disablement was symbolized by a correlation between her internal state of panic, and the disorder in the world outside. Her 'self-theory' contained a sense of vulnerability in the relationship between herself and the social world. In an attempt to mitigate this Mrs Fields had developed strategies whose essential purpose was encapsulated in the phrases: 'just-in-casing' and 'taking your time'. The former referred to her work at maintaining a level of tidiness and cleanliness in the home when she was feeling well so that things would not collapse completely when she was ill. The latter referred to an attitude required in doing things which involved calm determination and simple resignation when things proved impossible to do.

Mrs Fields was engaged in the development of 'coping strategies', where the term 'coping' refers to '... action directed at the resolution or mitigation of a problematic situation' (Ray, Lindop and Gibson 1982: 385), and 'strategy' implies 'the presence of conscious and rational decisions involving a long-term perspective' (Crow 1989: 19). These strategies allowed her to postpone chaos. However, further analysis of the interview transcript revealed a vulnerability and a sense of urgency informing these strategies which indicated that they were part of a deeper pursuit – the pursuit of virtue – the style of which suggests a particular view of society and her place within it. This pursuit revolved around three themes which, in different ways represent deep, interrelated connections between herself and society: dependence, uncleanliness, and indebtedness.

Being an encumbrance

Mrs Fields saw herself as being 'on her own'. By this she did not mean that she was without human contact but that, although now without a husband, the status of 'widow' did not confer special privileges legitimating her becoming 'an encumbrance' to anyone else. She regarded two sons living nearby as a potential resource, but insisted that they should be called upon only in extreme circumstances: 'They've their own lives to live, and as far as I can struggle I will do'. She was reluctant also to accept help from the statutory services, emphasizing that it 'wouldn't be fair' to take something that somebody worse off than herself might need. This was in contrast to her unabashed reliance on the health service for treatment of her disease, presumably because the disease was something over which she could not exert personal control however hard she tried. Moreover, while treatment of her disease was seen as a prerequisite for independence, human services intervention, in relation to self-care activities for example, might undermine it:

> 'Both girls (physical therapists) were about thirty, and I felt a bit embarrassed because I had to phone them and say "I want a bath, can you come down?". It was only for the sake of them coming in and helping me get down in the water, I was alright then. I thought I'd have to do something about this, and we had a look round and I said to her, "I'll tell you what I could do with, a bath-seat, but I want an adjustable one". So I got one of those and it's smashing. With that I've got independence. I can go up and have a bath when I want, you know, without asking anybody.'

There was a sense in which precisely because of the success of her coping strategies Mrs Fields felt all the more threatened by those areas of life involving other people over which control could not be assured. The bath-seat gave her control: 'You see, I can just go upstairs and run that bath anytime. I'm not worried about anybody, I could be there all afternoon and be quite happy with the fact that I've done it myself'.

The silence of the mechanical device was preferable to having to ask someone to help with self-care activities, even someone paid to do so. To say you are dependent on a thing – a walking stick or a drug – has a different connotation from being dependent on a person. It is irksome to be unable to get about without a stick, but it is much more inconvenient to have to wait for someone to come and take you out, and thereby feel that you are also constraining their lives as well (Williams 1987). Furthermore, dependence upon the kindness of a neighbour or the charity of a voluntary body has a different quality to dependence on the State. In this regard the welfare state has costs and benefits. Many people enjoy the immediacy of charitable giving but as Ignatieff notes in reflecting on his perception of the elderly in Western society:

> The mediated quality of our relationship seems necessary to both of us. They are dependent on the State, not upon me, and we are both glad of it. Yet I am also aware of how this mediation walls us off from each other. We are responsible for each other, but we are not responsible to each other.
>
> (Ignatieff 1984: 10)

While dependence upon a device may be upsetting because it exists as a constant reminder of disablement, it avoids the complications of reciprocity. Being dependent on another person creates a feeling of indebtedness which does not exist in relation to an object: 'I used to wonder what they think having to be tied to come round here and get me in the bath and get me out'. Furthermore, the bath-seat had particular importance because it permitted her to remain private in relation to an area of life where this is expected, and in relation to a set of activities of daily living competent performance of which is regarded as fundamental to social life.

The significance of uncleanliness

Anxiety about dirt and hygiene figures strongly in Mrs Fields's account, and was linked up with her desire to be independent and to do things in her own time:

> 'At least I'm independent. I can dress myself, I can wash myself, I clean up, to an extent, you know. I'm satisfied, I'm happy, it's my home, and that's it.'

This cluster of statements about self-mastery and the relationship between independence in self-care and personal happiness, expresses some powerful and closely related sentiments. A moment later she said: 'You know, things are not piling up – this is dirty and that's dirty – I just do it in my own time and I'm comfortable'. The implication here is that the control over time implied by the strategies referred to earlier, is made manifest in her dealing with dirty things around her. Dirt in the domestic milieu means that her strategies have failed, and this failure represents a loss of control over her environment. As Douglas has argued: 'Dirt offends against order. Eliminating it is not a negative movement, but a positive effort to organize the environment' (Douglas 1966: 2). Dirty things piling up are a sign of individual loss of control and social disorder and cleaning is part of a wider attempt to construct order within the life-world. Within this symbolic-interactive process the idea that other people might see her as dirty would be profoundly threatening:

> 'The other week, the district nurse came running in saying, "Do you mind if I use your toilet?" Now the first thought in my mind was "She's a nurse, they're particular, she wouldn't ask to go to my toilet if I was dirty". You know, you think you've achieved something. I know it may sound simple to you, but it's not. That was something important. She can't think I'm careless, and she's not frightened of touching anything in the house.'

Dirt was a symbol not only of disorder and loss of control but also of carelessness – a failure to discharge certain duties in the relationship between the person and the environment. It was important for Mrs Fields to be seen to be clean especially at those points where private spaces are opened to the public scrutiny of official strangers. Person and environment become fused within a metaphorical elaboration of the significance of dirt in which virtue means keeping one's house in order, and this is expressed through the performance of activities concerned with bodily and environmental hygiene.

One of the important points about virtue, however, is that it involves striving for the mean between deficiency and excess (Bambrough 1963) and between activity and rest (Berki, 1977). In the context of chronic illness this is particularly important because the sufferer is confronted with the competing demands of physiological and social imperatives (Wiener 1975). This dilemma was apparent when Mrs Fields said:

> 'I'm not so posh ... but I'm comfortable. If anyone comes along and they don't like it ... what can I do about it? I'm fortunate to keep it as straight as it is. If somebody's coming they take me as I am because doing too much I could cause myself a flare-up? Why should I do it to cover something up. They must come in and find me as I am day to day, which is right.'

There was clearly a tension in this recognition of her own physical limitations on the one hand, and her need, on the other, to conduct herself in such a way that her virtuousness would be acknowledged. She could struggle to display cleanliness and respectability to others but there was no guarantee that they would in turn appreciate the fragility of this reality. Being dirty, and the fear about what inferences might be drawn by others from that fact, was clearly a major threat to Mrs Fields's sense of identity: 'I used to worry that people would think I was getting old, and if I started getting dirty ...'. What was the source of this worry?

> 'Well, the thought of "hasn't she let herself go" and "she's not clean", that kind of thing which ... if you're poor you can be clean. I was thinking that it wasn't through any fault of my own, it was just that I wasn't capable of doing it.'

This final passage relating to the issue of dirt contains several key terms which mark aspects of the respondent's relations to society and history and point to the cohesiveness of her identity. Hasn't she let herself go! – you can almost hear the patronizing tones of neighbours and professionals. Although Mrs Fields had not herself lived through the Poor Laws, she was old enough to have memories stretching back to before the setting up of the welfare state and the National Health Service, and the juxtaposition of references to cleanliness and poverty, desert and blame, alongside disablement, forms a coherent expression of fear – the fear of pauperism and stigma. In this context, the fact that she was disabled or 'not capable' rather than reprehensible was very important because:

> The connection between disability and deception meant that the very category of disability was developed to incorporate a mechanism for distinguishing the genuine from the artificial.
>
> (Stone 1984: 32)

Dirt could be interpreted by others as meaning not simply that she was in fact ageing, but that her response to illness and ageing was weak and therefore blameworthy. She was letting herself go; it was her fault. She wanted people to understand that she was genuinely disabled, and that any 'failings' were caused by things outside her control. Moreover, her reason for believing that others might interpret the signs in this way was linked to another important fact about her life: 'Well, you know, because Albert (her late husband) wasn't here and all that business, and that I just couldn't care less. I didn't want anybody to get that impression. I still wanted that independence'.

Regardless of the actual relationship between her bereavement and her response to disablement, she was concerned about the extent to which people might regard signs of dirt as being to do with the effects of loss rather than anything else. Mrs Fields felt that other people might account for her carelessness and lack of hygiene in terms of the distortions of grief rather than physical incapacity. In the light of all this, the pursuit of virtue, in the form of cleanliness and control, was designed more to deal with a social context in which her actions would be interpreted rather than with her own specific disabilities.

The avoidance of debt

I have already indicated that some anxiety about poverty seemed to exist alongside her desire for independence. In the light of the fact that money and wealth are not only necessary to independence in our society but also symbols of autonomy, and that financial difficulties increase in the lives of people with disabilities (Martin and White 1988), it is interesting to note the place given over to discussion about money in Mrs Fields's account of her life with arthritis. Moreover, money is significant because it is critical to the maintenance of relationships between individuals and the wider society.

In the context of a discussion about whether 'worry' made her arthritis more likely to flare up she told me:

> 'Well ... I don't know why I should say this. I had money but it's tied up. You see, when my husband died, I invested his money for three years,

> which is till next year. So this year has been hard. You see, the first year I had a bit of money, this year, with bills and one thing and another ... and I'm stupid, I panic. I think it's the end of the world because I can't just go out and pay it straight away. I mean, it's no laughing matter if you've got rates, electric, gas and telephone bills all at the same time.'

A bill represents something owed to another person or agency in society. Although it may be payable to an individual, the expectation that it will be paid is social, and where that expectation is not met sanctions may be forthcoming. It represents a legitimate claim by one party on another for goods received or services rendered, and until the bill is paid the person is in a state of debt which, in the extreme, can be a very public state. To be in debt is to have ones virtue questioned in a profound way. In the context of Mrs Field's account, being in debt, like being dirty or untidy, could be taken to mean that she was careless, or that she was letting herself go; that she was allowing her life to slip. Increasingly, under the influence of 'Thatcherism', being able to look after money is seen as the defining characteristic of the competent human being.

Mrs Fields launched into a lengthy monologue on the details of bills, budgets, investment and interest. She felt suffocated by it:

> '... it was a mountain and I was at the bottom of it. I could pay one but there was three left, and if I paid them three what about my rates. I was thinking would I have a home and all that business... . If the 'phone rang I thought "I bet its connected with that bill".'

Dependence and the concern about being in debt were tied into the importance of being clean through the concrete need for a bath-seat. In a sense, within her account, the bath-seat provided the symbolic centre of all the anxieties and worries which have been described.

> 'The occupational therapist told me I could have the bath-seat through the social services. I said "No, how much are they to buy?" I think she said they were about four or five pounds. So I thought "I'll pay for it". Now it's mine. Nobody's coming knocking at the door saying "Have you finished with that?" It's mine, I can go up and use it when I want.'

The knock at the door, the inquiries into the condition of the appliance; the gas board telephoning about an unpaid bill; the neighbours whispering about her state of mind: all these involuntary interchanges with society represent a threat to autonomy, and this perceived threat drew Mrs Fields into urgent activity in pursuit of virtue. From the perspective of clinical medicine and rehabilitation she was 'coping well'. However, the very control she managed to sustain over her mundane activities and the immediate milieu revealed more starkly those areas over which control was impossible because they involved powerful external agencies, and served to underline the Durkheimian paradox of modern society in which the individual 'whilst becoming ever more autonomous, depends ever more closely upon society' (Durkheim 1984: 7).

CHRONIC ILLNESS AND EVERYDAY LIFE

The general prescriptions provided by professionals for people with chronic illness may be resisted, forgotten or ignored, both because they are too complicated and therefore difficult to integrate into the flux of daily life, and because they rest upon a set of presumptions about the meaning and significance of illness that are not wholly shared by the patient (Williams and Wood 1986). In a society in which 'self-control' is an important value, chronic illness represents a loss of control both because of the effects of the illness itself on the performance of daily activities, through the impact upon normal patterns of interdependence (Williams 1987), and because the person is expected to defer to the medical profession in the interests of health. Increasingly, however, the establishment of 'self-efficacy' in the sometimes life-long process of rehabilitation is reflected in self-management programmes for arthritis patients (Lorig *et al.* 1989). Faced with the facts of the ineffectiveness of medicine in treating chronic illness, and in the context of a resurgent belief in the sovereignty of the individual consumer and citizen, the 'moral life' may mean a life without doctors and their drugs, or making judicious use of them.

In the case of Mrs Fields we have seen how the issue of personal control over her life was important at a number of different levels. At the level of bodily integrity she sustained control to a great extent by following doctors' orders: in this she was an exemplary patient. In the self-management of disability, too, her attitude to the relations of time, activity and social support suggested personal adaptability and strategic good sense; and at this level the good life entailed doing as much as she could for herself in her own time. However, everyday life consists not just of the daily activities performed within known milieux, but also the structures within which those activities take the forms they do, and the representation of the force of those structures within our lives. It is in terms of such representations that we perceive our own activities as appropriate to the kind of people we take ourselves to be.

If we are to comprehend more fully what Antonovsky (1979) referred to as the sense of coherence that informs or fails to inform people's responses to difficult situations, then we have to recognize that the expressive terms people use cannot be reduced to instrumental terms of 'adjustment' and 'adaptation'. These concepts, staple components of the rehabilitation literature, tend to be ethically judgemental because they are unrelated to the context of the moral life of the person concerned. In order to avoid the pitfalls of judgement, we need to see coping strategies as moral practices where:

> a moral practice is, in part, a language of self-enactment; that is, a language in which conduct may be recognized in terms of its 'virtue' and an agent may recognize himself in terms of his 'virtuousness'
>
> (Oakeshott 1975: 75)

This notion of a moral practice is important because it helps to point to a source of tension in the experience of chronic illness. Terms such as adaptation, adjustment and coping refer to a world of contingency, the everyday world in which the individual interacts with others and experiences successes and failures. What we see in Mrs Fields's pursuit of virtue, however, is an attempt to enact a story about herself as she wishes to be understood, regardless of whether the enactment is the optimum way for her to proceed in the given circumstances. In this sense, my respondent made strategic uses of narrative to present herself as a person of a certain sort (Riessman 1990), and my analysis of her account of her life can be seen to include the cognitive, strategic and stylistic elements that Bury (1991) has recently advised us to distinguish.

The reality of life for most disabled people is not the heroic overcoming of dramatic obstacles, but the daily struggle with the mundane activities through which identity is expressed and confirmed: 'mundane activities are significant simply because they are mundane' (Locker 1983: 95). These activities need to be seen as not merely instrumental manipulations of the environment, but moral practices, expressing preferred styles of adaptation (Radley 1989) through which individuals enact themselves. This is not a matter of people denying or accepting the fact of illness, but of continuing to express themselves through the medium of their everyday activities (Cornwell 1984). It is this that underlies many of the statements people make about their responses to illness: 'Sometimes you wonder if you're being soft'; and 'people can make themselves be crippled by giving in to it'. If such sentiments are not related to an individual's social and narrative context (Williams 1989), they can be turned back on the person as judgements on their 'attitudes'.

The respondents in my work seemed to employ sets of vocabularies in terms of which their right and proper attitudes were expressed. 'He's always been a fighter', said one women of her arthritic husband, as if she wanted to convince herself as well as me that there was nothing shameful or blameworthy about his condition. The woman whose life we have already examined in some detail also said: '... if you're not willing to fight, it will want to overtake you altogether. That's no game at all'. Another said: 'If I were to say "Oh, I can't do this" and "This is getting me down" and "Well, I'll have to give in", I think that attitude is all wrong, with anything though, not just with this'. Such postures are echoed in actions which, in the context of chronic illness, attain great symbolic significance. One woman said: 'I think if you sit in a chair and say 'I've got (arthritis)' that's the end' and, in the same vein, a male respondent told me: 'I think you have got to fight .... If you are going to get into bed that is the end of it, that is my own feeling whether it is true or false'. In this way, 'sitting' and 'lying down' were doing far more than designating physical positions.

The accounts and actions through which virtue is displayed are not simply matters of individual motive because the contents of a person's mental life include the ideologies and belief-systems predominant in his or her society (Billig 1982). In other words, an individual's self-theory is a social theory. The pursuit of virtue is a component in the 'micro-politics' of everyday life:

> .... whenever somebody says 'human nature being what it is we have to do this or that'; whenever there is a sigh: 'this is the way of the world isn't it?'; whenever someone says that something or other is 'just not fit for human beings' or that this or that is 'not the proper way of doings things'; or whenever a man cries out: 'we all want to be happy don't we?'. Statements like this are nothing else but implicit or embryonic forms of political philosophy, condensed instances of political wisdom.
>
> (Berki 1977: 10)

The conflicts and tensions exhibited in the pursuit of virtue in particular cases can only be understood in relation to the wider social and historical settings through which someone has passed and in which they now live. Political thought, in this sense, is not something that exists only in books or parliaments, it is a constitutive part of the self-theories in terms of which individuals appraise and organize their everyday lives:

> What a person will be capable of will depend in part on the particular form of generic self-theory they acquire, because it is in terms of that theory that they will construe themselves as more or less autonomous, determined and so on.
>
> (Harré 1983: 102)

At the heart of everyday life is the interdependency of person and society (Wright, 1985). The vocabulary of fighting is part of a language of self-enactment through which virtue is displayed, but the forms it takes in a given instance are connected to concrete biographical experiences. Drawing on his personal knowledge of war, for example, one man said that you have to 'copy' from one experience to another: 'you survived in the (army) and you'll survive this'. The fact that arthritis is a disease does not exclude it also being a form of adversity; but in order to see this you have to take the 'patient's viewpoint' very seriously indeed; something most clinicians find difficult.

CONCLUSION

The modern vogue is to argue for the return of as many utilities and services as possible to the market in the belief that herein lies the fastest freeway to economic prosperity and individual liberty. However, the danger of a romance with individualism at a time of economic stringency in Western societies is the legitimation of inequality and neglect. In recent years arguments for greater consumer sovereignty and independence in relation to welfare systems have come, not only from politicians, but also from many disabled people who regard themselves as prisoners of the welfare state and dupes of the 'caring' professionals within it (De Jong 1979). I have argued elsewhere that this somewhat oversimplifies the situation for the vast majority of disabled people (Williams 1983, 1988). Independence is an important idea, but people overlook how much its reality depends upon the many resources an individual collects through his or her history, and upon the power structures which determine the way in which resources are distributed and made available.

It would be wrong to view the quality of people's daily life experiences as being in some unidirectional way determined by class position, gender relations, or social conditions in general. However, society certainly constrains people in all sorts of ways and, as I have tried to show in the case-study, these can be so subtle that an individual would not recognize them as socially imposed constraints at all. However, the point being made is that there is far more to coping with chronic illness than the instrumental self-management of symptoms; and, through the case-study, I have shown apparently disparate elements of biographical experience being drawn together as interconnected influences on the experience of chronic arthritis. This is important because: '... the unity of a virtue in someone's life is intelligible only as a characteristic of a unitary life, a life that can be conceived and evaluated as a whole' (Macintyre, 1981: 191).

In the case-study, independence in self-care, cleanliness, and solvency were clearly virtues which were held together within Mrs Fields's life as a unity; and while her specific disabilities could be dealt with in her own time and on her own terms, the threat to these virtues in her life came from society and drew her into a process of self-enactment through which potentially damaging evaluations could be resisted. The disadvantages relating to her arthritis were less the direct effects of her disease and more the product of her interaction with the social and physical world. Coping with a problematic physical condition, such as arthritis, involves coping with things other than the problematic condition itself.

What I have demonstrated in a modest and limited way through the case study is that living with chronic illness is a complex social process, and while individuals express a concern with responsibility and independence they recognize also that society and culture contain powerful forces determining the extent to which those qualities are able to emerge in an individual life. While disabilities may require individuals to develop certain strategies, the importance these strategies assume may depend far more on the nature of society and the individual's perceptions of their place in it.

ACKNOWLEDGEMENTS

The work on which this chapter is based was undertaken while the author was medical sociologist with the Arthritis and Rheumatism Council's Epidemiology Research Unit at the University of Manchester. The paper benefited from the pertinent comments of Philip Wood, but the author alone is responsible for the remaining inadequacies.

REFERENCES

Anderson, R. and Bury, M. (eds) (1988) *Living with Chronic Illness: the Experience of Patients and their Families*, London: Unwin Hyman.

Antonovsky, A. (1979) *Health, Stress and Coping*, Ohio: Jossey-Bass.

Bambrough, R. (1963) *The Philosophy of Aristotle*, Mentor: New American Library.

Berki, R. (1977) *An Introduction to Political Philosophy*, London: Dent.

Billig, M. (1982) *Ideology and Social Psychology*, Oxford: Blackwell.

Bury, M. (1991) 'The sociology of chronic illness: a review of research and prospects', *Sociology of Health and Illness* 13: 451–68.

Conrad, P. (1987) 'The experience of illness: recent and new directions', in J.A. Roth and P. Conrad (eds) *Research in the Sociology of Health Care, vol. 6, The Experience and Management of Chronic Illness*, Greenwich, Connecticut: JAI Press Inc.

Corbin, J. and Strauss, A. (1987) 'Accompaniments of chronic illness: changes in body, self, biography, and biographical time', in J.A. Roth and P. Conrad (eds) *Research in the Sociology of Health Care, vol. 6, The Experience and Management of Chronic Illness*, Greenwich, Connecticut: JAI Press Inc.

Cornwell, J. (1984) *Hard-Earned Lives: Accounts of Health and Illness from East London*, London: Tavistock Publications.

Crow, G. (1989) 'The use of the concept of "strategy" in recent sociological literature', *Sociology* 23: 1–24.

De Jong, G. (1979) *The Movement for Independent Living: Origins, Ideology, and Implications for Disability Research*, UCIR, Michigan State University.

Douglas, M. (1966) *Purity and Danger*, London: Routledge & Kegan Paul.

Durkheim, E. (1984) *The Division of Labour in Society* (originally 1893), London: Macmillan.

Gilsenan, M. (1989) 'Word of honour', in R. Grillo (ed.) *Social Anthropology and the Politics of Language, Sociological Review Monograph 36*, London: Routledge.

Gouldner, A. (1971) *The Coming Crisis of Western Sociology*, London: Heinemann.

Hall, S. (1988) *The Hard Road to Renewal: Thatcherism and the Crisis of the Left*, London: Verso.

Harré, R. (1983) *Personal Being: A Theory for Individual Psychology*, Oxford: Blackwell.

Heller, A. (1984) *Everyday Life*, London: Routledge & Kegan Paul.

Ignatieff, M. (1984) *The Needs of Strangers*, London: Chatto & Windus.

Illsley, R. (1981) 'Problems of dependency groups: the care of the elderly, the handicapped, and the chronically ill', in *Social Science and Medicine*, 15A: 327–32.

Locker, D. (1983) *Disability and Disadvantage: the Consequences of Chronic Illness*, London: Tavistock Publications.

Lorig, K., Chastain, R.L., Ung, E., Shoor, S. and Holman, H.R. (1989) Development and evaluation of a scale to measure perceived self-efficacy in people with arthritis', *Arthritis and Rheumatism* 32: 37–44.

Lukes, S. (1973) *Individualism*, Oxford: Basil Blackwell.

MacIntyre, A. (1981) *After Virtue: A Study in Moral Theory*, London: Duckworth.

Martin, J. and White, A. (1988) 'The Financial Circumstances of Disabled Adults Living in Private Households', *OPCS Surveys of Disability in Great Britain, Report 2*, London: Her Majesty's Stationery Office.

Mills, C.W. (1970) *The Sociological Imagination*, Harmondsworth: Penguin.

Oakeshott, M. (1975) *On Human Conduct*, Oxford: Clarendon Press.

Parker, J. and Mirrlees C. (1988) 'Welfare', in A.H. Halsey, *British Social Trends since 1900: a Guide to the Changing Social Structure of Britain*, London: Macmillan.

Radley, A. (1989) 'Style, discourse and constraint in adjustment to chronic illness', *Sociology of Health and Illness* 11: 231–52.

Ray, C., Lindop, J. and Gibson, S. (1982) 'The concept of coping', *Psychological Medicine* 12: 385–95.

Riessman, C.K. (1990) 'Strategic uses of narrative in the presentation of self and illness: a research note', *Social Science and Medicine* 30: 1195–200.

Rodmell, S. and Watt, A. (1986) *The Politics of Health Education: Raising the Issues*, London: Routledge & Kegan Paul.

Runciman, W.G. (1983) *Treatise on Social Theory (vol. 1), The Methodology of Social Theory*, Cambridge: Cambridge University Press.

Sennett, R. and Cobb, J. (1973) *The Hidden Injuries of Class*, New York: Vintage Books.

Skidelsky, R. (ed.) (1988) *Thatcherism*, London: Chatto & Windus.

Stone, D. (1984) *The Disabled State*, London: Macmillan.

Taylor, C. (1985) *Human Agency and Language. Philosophical Papers, Vol. 1*, Cambridge: Cambridge University Press.

Taylor-Gooby, P. (1987) 'Citizenship and welfare', in R. Jowell, S. Witherspoon and L Brook (eds) *British Social Attitudes: the 1987 Report*, Aldershot: Gower.

Wear, A. (1985) 'Puritan perceptions of illness in seventeenth century England', in R. Porter (ed.) *Patients and Practitioners: Lay Perceptions of Medicine in Pre-Industrial Society*, Cambridge: Cambridge University Press.

Weber, M. (1976) *The Protestant Ethic and the Spirit of Capitalism*, London: Counterpoint, Unwin Paperbacks.

West, P., Illsley, R. and Kelman, H. (1984) 'Public preferences for the care of dependency groups', *Social Science and Medicine* 18: 287–95.

Wiener, C. (1975) 'The burden of rheumatoid arthritis: tolerating the uncertainty', *Social Science and Medicine*, 9: 97–104.

Williams, G.H. (1983) 'The movement for independent living: an evaluation and critique', *Social Science and Medicine* 17: 1003–10.

Williams, G.H. (1987) 'Disablement and the social context of daily activity', *International Disability Studies* 9: 97–102.

Williams, G.H. (1988) 'Independent living: rolling back the frontiers of the State?', *Disability Studies Quarterly* Spring: 50–4.

Williams, G.H. (1989) 'The genesis of chronic illness: narrative reconstruction', in P. Brown (ed.) *Perspectives in Medical Sociology*, Belmont: Wadsworth.

Williams, G.H. and Wood, P.H.N. (1986) 'Common-sense beliefs about illness: a mediating role for the doctor', *The Lancet*, 11: 1435–37.

Wright, P. (1985) *On Living in an Old Country: The National Past in Contemporary Britain*, London: Verso.

6 The role of metaphor in adjustment to chronic illness

Alan Radley

There is now a growing literature on the ways that people live with and adjust to chronic illnesses of various kinds (for reviews, see Anderson and Bury 1988; Bury 1991; Roth and Conrad 1987). To suffer from a chronic illness is to be faced with a situation in which, depending upon the nature of the disease, people continue to live a more or less normal existence. One of the key directions in research to date has addressed the question of the basic strategies people use in order that they might live as normal a life as possible (Strauss 1975; Corbin and Strauss 1987). The implied stigma of illness requires that some sufferers employ a range of tactics either to hide or to modify differences, so that they might be accepted as fully capable participants in social life. To fall short of such acceptance, either through the nature of the disease manifestations (e.g. rectal cancer [MacDonald 1988]) or through being judged as failing to bear one's illness properly, is to risk being deemed 'less of a person'. The chronically ill are subject to cultural expectations that, in their evaluation of the personal and social status of the afflicted, can be said to be the expression of a public morality.

This focus upon normalization is consistent with the conceptualization of illness as a form of biographical disruption (Bury 1982). This view draws attention to chronic illness as a critical situation calling for an answer to the question, 'what is going on here?'. The uncertainty that many patients feel is something that is addressed in terms of their personal situation and their stock of common knowledge about health and illness. One way of making sense of one's fate as a sick person is through what has been termed 'narrative reconstruction' (Williams 1984). For the sick person not only needs to appear normal to others, but also to make sense of his or her life in the context of a continuing and perhaps worsening disability. One role of such a narrative is to reconstruct the course of one's life so that it accommodates the illness by providing it with a 'genesis'. Williams used this term to reveal how such narratives are not merely a record of private events, but can expand into a more general critique of the political and institutional situation of the persons concerned. In this way a convincing account of one's normality (social competence) and a reasonable account of one's illness situation are established in what has been termed 'the merging of public morality and private fate' (Gerhardt 1989: 214).

These comments suggest that we should view adjustment to chronic illness as more than the functional adaptation of an ailing body to the demands of a healthy society (Alonzo 1979), and more than the telling of stories by patients about the course of the illness itself (Robinson 1990). The illness experience is not only the precipitating feature in the person's reconstruction of events, but is also part of the claim that the person makes about his or her standpoint in the world of health. Not only must the chronically ill account for their condition (to repair biographical disruption) and arrange the detail of their lives (to avoid stigma): they must also legitimate their actions in a way that says that they are doing their best and are therefore free from moral condemnation by others (Voysey 1975).

There are two features of this problem to which I shall pay special attention in this chapter. One is the way in which illness itself can become a window on the world of health, becoming a context or frame within which the remainder of the person's life can be evaluated and approached. The other is the way in which adjustment to illness, if it is to be self-legitimating, needs to have a certain communicative structure. This structure is most readily seen as metaphor, or rather as one kind of metaphor among several that are used by patients to give expressive form to their condition.

LITERAL AND METAPHORIC RESPONSES TO ILLNESS

There are two meanings that can be given to the word metaphor when speaking of how sick people reconstrue their lives. First, the way that individuals use figures of speech in how they represent their illness to themselves and to others, and second the way that certain adjustments involve a re-figuration of the subject in his or her dealings with other people. The first aspect is one with which, I think, we are more familiar; the use of language to represent a change in situation. The second, being less apparent, invites a deeper scrutiny of the way that metaphor is used by people in coming to terms with illness that is either chronic, or serious or both.

One example of the use of metaphor as a way of constructing 'cognitively and linguistically' the course of illness has been given by Duval (1984). She describes how a patient used metaphorical expressions to reconcile conflicts surrounding a diagnosis of multiple sclerosis, first denying the implications of the disease (references to 'living in a house with stairs') while later acceding to the possibilities of a negative prognosis (references to herself as 'becoming like a vegetable'). The use of figurative language to capture fleeting experiences, particularly in cases where the medical diagnosis is unclear or the prognosis uncertain, has been seen as having either positive (Taussig 1980) or negative consequences (Sontag 1979). What might be called the evaluative potential of metaphor in formulating illness experience is tied up with differing views about the value of medical terminology in the patient's attempt to come to terms with a chronic condition and all that this implies (Bury 1982; Taussig 1980).

It is an open question as to the conditions which foster the use of metaphoric thinking in these circumstances and the consequences of so doing. At one level, as we shall see below, all thinking is shot through with metaphor, so that the question of when it is used by patients becomes redundant. However, the issue is wider than the use of figurative language alone and it is to this wider concern that I now turn.

In a description of a group of cardiac patients who underwent surgery for their condition, I drew attention to different forms of adjustment to coronary disease, and to how these can be comprehended within the context of the patient's conjugal relationship and wider social network (Radley 1988). On the basis of those findings, it is possible to draw out a distinction in the way that patients described their situation that bears upon the question of metaphor in the experience of chronic disease. On the one hand were patients who responded to their condition by countering directly the intrusions of the disease, opposing these in order to minimize symptoms and to maximize normal life as far as possible. This outlook is one that dismisses the inactivity that has been said to commit the person to sickness through a changed relationship to society (Herzlich 1973). When formulated by the person concerned as a definite approach to dealing with disease, it can appear as follows:

> 'I'm too strong a character to let it. It's as simple as that. I won't let anything beat me, basically. In any sphere, I hate not to do my own thing and make a success of it. I will not be beaten by illness and related things. Nobody beats me.'

Patients who responded by opposing their illness in this way seemed to be engaged in a fight in which heart disease took on a literal quality, something with which to wrestle. In contrast were individuals who seemed to use the illness experience as a way of re-orienting themselves, working their way around limitations in order to accommodate the implications of coronary disease. For example, one cardiac patient said:

> 'There's a point at which you find a crossroads perhaps but you take another direction, you change your way of life but that way of life might not necessarily be impoverished for being different.'

This accommodation involved patients in treating the symptoms and the consequent limitations upon their life as if they were indications of a new order that offered different, though not necessarily inferior opportunities for the future. Their approach to illness had a figural quality, that transformed symptoms from signs with which they had to deal to symbols allowing them to conceive of change. This approach to illness has been noted before, not least by authors wishing to draw attention to the positive outcomes accompanying this perspective (Sacks 1982).

It is this difference between the literal and the figurative in patients' styles of adjustment that forms the focus for the remainder of this chapter. It needs to be said that, in pointing up this distinction, I am not attempting an empirical exercise, saying which patients adjust in which way and with what result. Instead, the argument is based upon a distinction that, having arisen out of empirical research, is here being elevated to an ideal form. It can then serve as a vehicle for discussing how such a difference matters in how we conceptualize the problem of adjustment to serious illness. However, before addressing this problem directly I need first to say something about metaphor and how others have analysed it.

SOME IDEAS ABOUT METAPHOR

There is a wide appreciation of the use of metaphor in everyday life (for a review, see Mair 1977). Metaphors have been described as the vital means by which people discover and create the realities of their world, as well as being seen as limitations of thought, as when we mistake the label for the thing being indicated.

The idea that metaphor is just a matter of comparison of one thing in terms of another is a view criticized as being far too limited (Barbour 1974). For example, the phrase 'he had the strength of a lion' can be explained in terms of a comparison of the physical strength of men and lions, but to do so is to empty the metaphor of its significance. What makes a metaphor meaningful is the way in which one aspect of experience is invigorated by another. In the previous example we do not see the man as being just of a particular degree of strength, that could have been expressed in horsepower (a 'dead metaphor'), but having a quality that comes from his being appreciated in terms of lions and their world. The power of metaphor is always lost if we attempt the reduction of one feature to the other or see it as mere comparison. For it is not just the similarity between the things compared that is important but also the difference. What allows the appreciation of metaphor rather than plain comparison is the difference between the terms that cannot be accounted for. Men are not lions even when their strength invites the comparison, any more than they are donkeys when their stupidity suggests that they be seen in this alternative way. The significance lies in the simultaneous appreciation of this similarity-difference identity.

The point about metaphor is that both its principal and subsidiary subjects are transformed and yet preserved. To speak of one's illness as 'a crossroads' is not only to organize one's recovery in a particular way, but also to give all forms of crossing a symbolic value that they might not have had beforehand (Berggren 1962). And insofar as these other forms of crossing appear in what might be termed the 'healthy' aspects of a person's life (or biography), then they are reconstructed in relation to the domain of illness that they have come to symbolize. The import of the metaphor lies in this double transformation, which creates a new meaning out of the tension of the irreducible comparison mentioned already. A metaphor, therefore, is less a way of seeing how one thing is like another, than it is of reflecting one reality through another (Romanyshyn 1982). This reflection is a re-figuring of being ill, perhaps opening up avenues of action that previously could not be entertained. To reflect knowingly upon illness is also to intend to do so, to engage the world in such a way that it is transformed at those points where it is subtended by the metaphor. Taking a metaphoric attitude is therefore not a reflection upon the 'real' world once it *has* changed, but a reflection that *is* a kind of change in itself.

One further point needs to be made about metaphor. The reference to seeing one reality through another suggests not the use of isolated categories but entire 'domains of experience' (Lakoff and Johnson 1980). For example, the world of the cancer patient has been shown to be subject to metaphors that compare it with war and with malignancy (Sontag 1979). The argument here is that negative ideas drawn from other areas of life are imported into illness experience and create an unnecessary burden for the sick.

On the other hand, the world of illness as experienced by its sufferers can itself provide a vehicle for re-evaluating other domains of experience. (This relates to the point made above that both principal and subsidiary aspects of metaphor are preserved, transformed.) Significantly, the realm of bodily experience, so often made subsidiary or occluded in a world of words and abstractions, can become the way in which other aspects of life can be understood. Specifically, the salience of the body and of the symptoms associated with particular diseases can become signifiers of variations in daily life, e.g. the issue of 'balance' in the life of the sufferer from Parkinson's disease (Pinder 1988). Seeing how this might work more generally requires that we go back to some differences in the way that people adjust to illness. Using heart disease as the illustration, we can examine how metaphor can mean more than the use of words to describe one's condition or experience.

THE ROLE OF METAPHOR IN ADJUSTMENT TO ILLNESS

From what has been said so far, it is reasonable to conclude that all instances of chronic illness are likely to involve metaphoric thinking on the part of the people concerned. This is because they are confronted with the situation of having to live with their illness in a world of health. However, this does not mean that every individual uses metaphor in the same way or to the same degree.

In the previous section the distinction was made between patients who opposed coronary disease as if it were an entity and those who accommodated to it through a view based upon metaphor. Some elaboration on this distinction will show things to be not as simple as this division would first imply.

What I have called 'the literal view' was held mainly by patients who retained their lifestyle through minimizing symptoms and marginalizing their effects. One of the ways to do this was by referring to feelings as 'just being sore, not a pain', or coronary bypass surgery as being 'like having a boil removed from your neck'. The comparison of the features of heart disease with other lesser conditions, and their embedding in the projects of everyday life were ways to carry out this containment of perturbations to the normal way of life. This included what are essentially analogies, if not metaphors, in order to establish the ordinariness of their situation. Speaking of the heart as a pump is an example of such thinking; it particularizes and locates the disease at a stable point in the objective body.

One reason for seeing things in this way might be, as Sontag (1979) has suggested, that the mechanical metaphor implies that there is no responsibility, no disgrace in having the disease. In these cases, metaphor is used to describe not only the nature of the problem but also the kind of therapeutic relationship preferred. For example, coronary surgery was said by one patient to be like having your car serviced so that it will give you trouble-free motoring in the future.

We can, following Fernandez (1974), distinguish between the use of metaphor that likens blocked coronary arteries to furred-up pipes and that which indicates a different form to one's life in the light of illness. On the one hand is 'perspective metaphor', that works upon a predicate (like the heart, the artery) that is held clearly in mind. On the other, there is 'prescinding metaphor' that figures the abstract or the intangible in terms of something more concrete and specifiable in the predicate. Thus, one's attitude to illness is given form through it being reflected in terms of something tangible and specifiable, such as navigation. It is to the latter form of metaphor that I am referring when I speak of the accommodation of patient to illness.

For the cardiac patients who had accommodated to their heart disease, an integral part of using metaphor was the realization that their lives had changed irredeemably. To speak of 'keeping a balance' in one's activities or of 'being at the crossroads' included such a recognition. There was a self-consciousness in the way that such individuals spoke of the way that they monitored their activity levels, re-evaluated time spent at work, and took advantage of the time that being ill had forced upon them. The advantages of taking this line was that, whatever metaphor was used, the reconstruction of their illness gave them a position from which to handle the unpredictable events that related to the surgery for their condition.

The establishment of a new position involves the coupling of different domains of experience. This constitutes an affective movement of the subject, which has been claimed as one of the 'missions of metaphor' (Fernandez 1974). Fernandez calls this the movement of inchoate subjects into quality space. In this context it refers to the apprehension by the people concerned that a particular way of figuring their experience has made a significant difference, that it matters to them to engage their problems in this way. From the position of the outsider, it appears as a perspective through which the uncertainties of illness and the loose ends of the patient's biography are rendered sensible.

This positive movement contrasts most clearly with the situation of the heart patients who, treating illness only as a thing to be struggled against, were subject to its negative effects. At the point where everyday beliefs broke down, or were seriously invalidated by experience, people were confronted with the possibility that these were no longer sustainable truths. For these individuals there was only a narrowed and intensive effort to try to wrench back a near-normal existence. Put simply, the world that was 'really good' had become 'really bad'.

How might metaphor rescue this situation, or show a way out of this impasse? Romanyshyn (1982) offered an illustration that has a parallel with the unfairness felt by some individuals who fall prey to chronic disease.

A man has believed all his life in the triumph of justice but is one day wrongfully charged with murder. He is then faced with a contradiction (justice metes out injustice) which, treated at a literal level, is impossible to resolve. Then, out of this conflict emerges a sense of the 'blindness of justice'. This is a metaphoric appreciation in that the limited vision so figured indicates the human imperfection of which he has become a victim. Romanyshyn argues that this movement from mythic experience, through the struggle of literal contradiction to metaphoric realization is somehow therapeutic. While, in the context of chronic disease, this movement does not remove the illness situation, it might release the person from swinging between the twin poles of naive hope and naive despair. Such vacillation between these alternatives is, in fact, a perfect description of the situation of patients who struggled fruitlessly against their heart disease in what has been termed a literal fashion (Radley 1988).

I am not suggesting in this that the use of metaphor solves the problem of adjustment to illness, nor that it is restricted to a few people, or that it is a property of individuals taken separately. Indeed, Helman (1987) has suggested that the fate of the heart attack victim in Western society is constituted within an ideology that poses the individual as a figure of moral ambiguity. The contradictions inherent in the model of the coronary-prone individual (whose restless ambition is both valued and censured) set a paradox within which the literal struggle described above, and its implications for the body, can be understood (Radley 1984). More to the point, however, is Helman's suggestion that adjustment to a heart attack, which involves the victim in renouncing his [sic] prior lifestyle, be viewed as a resolution of this moral paradox. The public's beliefs about heart disease are extended through the discourse on stress (Pollock 1988), which provides a framework that both specifies and leaves people open to the contradictions embraced within its mythology.

Seen in this way, the use of metaphor in adjustment to illness is insufficiently understood as a cognitive or even as an individual affair. Nor, I would add, is it adequately comprehended as an aspect of a socio-linguistic system, for the simple reason that the figuration of the life-world involves the body. This is not a reference to the supposed reality of bodily feelings, but to the fact that the resolution of the demands of culture and of symptoms, the merging of public morality and private fate, finds its place in the activity of the person concerned.

METAPHOR AND THE BODY

Metaphor is easiest to define in terms of language use. This does not mean, however, that it is restricted to what can be said in words. The idea of reflecting one domain of experience through another is a way of intending a meaning, engaging the world. The reflection of one domain through another is a subjective intention in the phenomenological sense, and in the realm of illness particularly it involves the cross-relation of bodily powers and experience. When we fall ill, our bodies are located as being, if not the site of trouble, then at least the point of disclosure that all is not well. However, this does not mean that the body suddenly takes on a significance that it did not have already; our lives are thoroughly embodied even as they are socially formed.

Lakoff and Johnson (1980) define 'domains of experience' as experiential gestalts or structured wholes. They are 'natural' in the sense of involving our bodies, our interactions with the physical environment and with other individuals. Appeals to naturalism always risk accusations of naive realism. For that reason it is essential to avoid the idea that metaphors are just linguistic devices for organizing the 'real' but diffuse experiences of an ailing body. Neither the world of health nor the world of illness is cut by such a line of cleavage.

The differences, already outlined, between patients who normalize and those who accommodate to illness are not merely distinctions in speech usage. They are also differences in the way that people use their bodies in everyday life (Murphy and Fischer 1983). Take for example a man in the cardiac sample who always insisted on digging his garden even though he knew it upset his wife. The act of digging can be seen as important because it signified to those around him the attitude that he took to his illness. It was not the only act of this kind, but it was readily specifiable as such. What might it be meant to convey? That he was active? Certainly. That he was healthy? Only in part. For the digging was only salient in the context of his heart disease, something known to his family and friends. Therefore, this action can be seen to stand for a relationship of the man to his illness and to the world of health. It said – perhaps more powerfully than words – that he refused the sick role in spite of the doctor having diagnosed him as having a serious illness. It becomes understandable in terms of his relationships to his wife and to his work, each one realized, respectively, in the way he could signify with bodily potentialities of sexuality and maleness.

In this example, the digging can be read as standing for the man's relationship to other areas of life, including his role as husband in the home and as someone still capable of doing a day's work if need be (he was a retired manual worker). This is a metonymic relationship in that the physical actions involved are also constituent 'parts' of other areas of life, which (were they to be put into words) might be described as benefiting from 'putting one's back into it' or 'getting stuck in'.

We can generalize from this illustration by seeing it as an example of the way that people frame their relationship to the worlds of health and illness simultaneously. In doing this, the point is made that the act (in this case, digging) says something about what the man is doing in relation to what others might expect of him. Insofar as there is then the implication of a distance between what is expected and what can be attained, then there is created a potential space for action. In this the person can evoke a response from others in making a claim to be a certain kind of person, in effect, through establishing a particular moral position.

'Framing' is another way of talking about metaphor in this context, as a way of reflecting one domain in terms of another. Bateson (1987) introduced this idea by reference to the way that animals signal play by nipping each other. The nip, in this case a metonym, is a modification of a bite. It signals play by saying something like, 'this nip which denotes a bite does not denote what a bite would normally denote'. Therefore, the nip signifies *both the absence and the presence* of the bite. It is part of a new code while also signifying the relationship between the domains of play and fighting. It is in this latter respect that it can be said to have a metaphoric function. (Wilden, 1972).

If we apply this idea to the digging of the cardiac patient, then this too can be seen as both symptomatic of a particular orientation and as a signifier of the intended relationship between the domains of health and illness for this individual. The act is doubly constituted as part of his way of life and as a sign through which might be grasped the tension of his working out of the relationship of illness and of health.

The points made about the irreducibility of metaphor apply here too. The man does not dig to say that he is cured – that his is a life of health. He digs to show that he can carry on in spite of his ailment. But more than this, he digs to reflect his relationship to his wife through a disregard of the dangers of bringing about a heart attack or indeed his own death. This example shows that metaphor does not merely link separate domains, but issues from an experience that is only subsequently apportioned to the realm of the body on the one hand, and to that of the social on the other. This specifiability of one's position, of how one lives with an illness like heart disease, is a linking of body and social world in a metaphor that is enacted as well as, or instead of, being said in words.

THE SCOPE FOR METAPHOR

The idea that metaphor might play a significant role in the construction of illness was given prominence by Susan Sontag (1979) in her book *Illness as Metaphor*. She made the argument that the sick continue to be the subject of 'punitive and sentimental fantasies' concocted about them and their condition. Applied especially to the chronic, intractable and sometime mysterious diseases such as tuberculosis, and more recently to cancer, the process of subjecting illnesses to figurative thinking has led to further moral judgements upon the sick. It is the way that healthy people use disease as a metaphor in their discourse that creates the lurid images that the sick must then continue to bear.

Sontag's point is that illness is not a metaphor, and she argues that the most truthful (and by implication, the healthiest) way of being ill is one purified of and resistant to metaphoric thinking. However, this seems to imply an understanding of illness in biomedical terms alone, once the mysteries surrounding disease have been extinguished by medical research. On this point, Sontag's analysis is limited and ultimately unhelpful, as it leads directly to an acceptance of the reification of disease, thus marginalizing the very attempts by the sick to express their illness experience (Scheper-Hughes and Lock 1986). The fact that these attempts employ cultural metaphors deemed to have negative as well as positive consequences is actually a reason to comprehend their workings, not to argue for their removal.

As has been pointed out elsewhere, Sontag's points about the work of metaphor are not restricted to diseases such as tuberculosis and cancer alone (Frankenberg 1986). While these might be the diseases about which there has been woven much figurative language in society, the use of metaphor by the sick extends to all kinds of illnesses. The reason for this is that there is a general requirement upon the sick to render their situation viable and comprehensible. In response to this, metaphor appears, in its various forms, to be one important means by which they might face up to this ongoing challenge.

One further point of difference should be mentioned. Sontag was referring to the way that images of illness are used by the healthy, whereas this chapter has addressed how a way of life touched by disease can be reconstrued from the position of the sick. Arguably, however, these are not quite separate issues, given that the power to figure, to construct metaphor, lies with the dominant domain, with the world of health.

Historical analysis of disease in society, and of the relationship of the sick to the healthy, shows these to be subject to transitions that provide a context within which the question of metaphor can be addressed. Herzlich and Pierret (1987) point out that:

> In all of these cases the reality and the image of the illness have ceased to be collective and have become those of an individual ailment. It is a *specific individual* who is sick, ...
>
> (1987: 49, emphasis in original)

They also show that, from the nineteenth century onward, it became important to have a labour force that could meet production needs. As a consequence, there was a linking of health with the capacity to work, so that illness became a social phenomenon. Ultimately,

> In the course of this double movement toward the individualization and socialization of illness, one new category has definitely emerged: *the sick*.
>
> (1987: 53, emphasis in original)

The emergence of the sick as a social category meant that there came with it the social perception of sick people as having an identity, something that they have to master, accept and employ in their dealings with other people. It is as part of this movement that we have sketched out a place for the use of metaphor by the chronically ill.

I want now to use Herzlich and Pierret's idea of the double movement toward individualization and socialization of illness to say something about the scope for using metaphor by people with chronic disease. Let us propose that this double movement is incorporated within the experience of all chronically sick individuals as the dilemma of having to resolve the demands of culture, of public morality, with the duty to one's individual health. (For example, among the cardiac patients some men spoke of having to refuse the demands of work in favour of their health; others worked extra hours in spite of a worsening condition to which they felt they ought to attend.) What we might call 'the tension of public morality versus private fate' reflects the potential space to which reference was made in terms of what is expected of the sick and what they can achieve. The resolution of the demands implicit in this potential is the person's way of bearing illness. My thesis is that the work of metaphor is part of this attempted resolution, its primary function being to give affective expression to experiences relating to matters of stigma, uncertainty, fear and pain.

We have already seen, however, that patients in the cardiac sample varied in how they used metaphor in the way that they adjusted to their condition. The main distinction drawn was between those who reconstructed their lives and those who used metaphor to retain their involvement in everyday life. One possibility might be that the 'double movement', the potential space is different for individuals in varying locations in the social structure. This would mean that the scope for using metaphor in the prescinding sense, as a way of re-figuring one's life, is not equally applicable to all. By this I mean the way that using a particular metaphor (of a 'prescinding' kind) organizes the uncertainties of illness so that people not only feel they have a grasp of their situation but have the greatest sense of self-determination.

In the cardiac study the difference between those who expressed or reported this scope and those that did not related to whether they held a white or blue collar job (Radley 1989). In particular, where individuals were forced to take early retirement, or where their employment allowed them greater opportunity for reorganizing their work, then they seemed (a) less subject to social demands about what they ought to be doing and, (b) more concerned to shape their own lives in future. For these patients, the use of metaphors that reconstructed their biographies seemed apposite and helpful. By contrast, where patients were employed in manual jobs, and hence felt more directly the need to maintain a body 'fit for work', then this ethic seemed to press on them strongly, so that their selves, in being bound up with work, mattered less as a focus for determining their fate. In the latter case, it was as if the demands of work and normal family life (public morality) was exercised more directly upon them. The potential for re-figuring life is small here; the discordance produced by disease exists, but is met with attempts at normalization, the use of metaphor that compares in order to conserve and to hold together existing structures.

By comparison, expressive metaphor that achieves affective movement re-constitutes the patient as a subject; that is, as someone who has the sense of power to signify about his or her illness condition. It may be that different ideologies provide the moral backing for claims of different kinds. These ideologies provide the 'public moralities' to which reference has already been made, upon which people draw in order to make sense of their fate and to legitimate their way of dealing with it. This would mean that the power to signify in this way does not lie with individuals alone, but with agencies and contexts that make available the ideas that people use to legitimate their way of dealing with suffering and spoiled ambitions (Voysey 1975).

Finally, this raises questions about when metaphor is employed and about the interpretation of accounts by researchers. People have a number of different explanations of health and illness and, it has been argued, they may employ these accounts in different ways depending upon context (Rogers 1991). Take for example the case of someone adjusting knowingly, a characteristic of metaphoric expression that was outlined earlier on. By speaking of oneself as a 'navigator' the style effectively announces itself. By this I mean that the understanding by the interviewer of what the patient is saying is contiguous with the researcher's apprehension of the metaphoric status of the term employed. In contrast, the man who said that heart surgery was like having a boil removed from his neck did not make this claim to a reconstruction of events. He was only concerned to draw out the similarities that restricted the operation's importance. What then becomes important is the literalness of this comparison. This, however, is something attributed by the researcher (e.g. the style of 'active-denial', Radley 1988) because of the differences that exist between the removal of boils and surgery to the cardiovascular system. That is, the use of metaphor, the drawing of perspectives is understood in relation to particular positions and motives that need to be comprehended in the context of the relationship of researcher to interviewee.

In effect, the statements that sick people make to interviewers have a double signification (Hall 1981) in that they are attempts, if not to articulate certain codes into a position of dominance, then at least to define the relation of their perspective to events as one of reality. This legitimation of how one speaks (and acts) is a communication seemingly in addition to the particular meanings that the person's account provides. Therefore, ways of bearing illness are constituted within modes of relationship that are encouraged, merely accepted or resisted as they are negotiated within the world of health. In conclusion, it can be said that the importance of examining metaphor in adjustment to chronic illness lies precisely in highlighting these different ways in which various experiences of sickness are given expressive form.

REFERENCES

Alonzo, A.A. (1979) 'Everyday illness behavior: A situational approach to health status deviations', *Social Science and Medicine* 13A: 397–404.

Anderson R. and Bury, M. (eds) (1988) *Living with Chronic Illness: the experience of patients and their families*, London: Unwin Hyman.

Barbour, I.G. (1974) *Myths, Models and Paradigms*, London: SCM Press.

Bateson, G. (1987) 'A theory of play and fantasy', in G. Bateson, *Steps to an Ecology of Mind*, London: Jason Aronson.

Berggren, D. (1962) 'The use and abuse of metaphor', *Review of Metaphysics* 16: 237–58.

Bury, M. (1982) 'Chronic illness as biographical disruption', *Sociology of Health and Illness* 4: 167–82.

Bury, M. (1991) 'The sociology of chronic illness: a review of research and prospects', *Sociology of Health and Illness* 13: 451–68.

Corbin, J. and Strauss, A.L. (1987) 'Accompaniments of chronic illness: changes in body, self, biography, and biographical time', in J.A. Roth and P. Conrad (eds) *Research in the Sociology of Health Care, vol. 6, The Experience and Management of Chronic Illness*, Greenwich, Connecticutt: JAI Press Inc.

Duval, M.L. (1984) 'Psychosocial metaphors of physical distress among MS patients', *Social Science and Medicine*, 19: 635–38.

Fernandez, J. (1974) 'The mission of metaphor in expressive culture' *Current Anthropology* 15: 119–45.

Frankenberg, R. (1986) 'Sickness as cultural performance: drama, trajectory, and pilgrimage. Root metaphors and the making social of disease', *International Journal of Health Services* 16: 603–26.

Gerhardt, U. (1989) *Ideas about Illness: an intellectual and political history of medical sociology*, London: Macmillan.

Hall, S. (1981) 'Notes on deconstructing "the popular" ', in R. Samuel (ed.) *People's History and Socialist Theory*, Boston: Routledge & Kegan Paul.

Helman, C.G. (1987) 'Heart disease and the cultural construction of time: the Type A Behaviour Pattern as a Western culture-bound syndrome', *Social Science and Medicine* 25: 969–79.

Herzlich, C. (1973) *Health and Illness: a social-psychological analysis*, London: Academic Press.

Herzlich, C. and Pierret, J. (1987) *Illness and Self in Society*, Baltimore: Johns Hopkins University Press. (Translated by E. Forster.)

Lakoff, G. and Johnson, M. (1980) *Metaphors We Live By*, Chicago: University of Chicago Press.

MacDonald, L. (1988) 'The experience of stigma: living with rectal cancer', in R. Anderson and M. Bury (eds) *Living with Chronic Illness: the experience of patients and their families*, London: Unwin Hyman.

Mair, J.M.M. (1977) 'Metaphors for living', in A.W. Landfield (ed.) *Nebraska Symposium on Motivation 1976*, Lincoln: University of Nebraska Press.

Murphy, M.A. and Fischer, C.T. (1983) 'Styles of living with low back injury: the continuity dimension', *Social Science and Medicine* 17: 291–7.

Pinder, R. (1988) 'Striking balances: living with Parkinson's Disease', in R. Anderson and M. Bury (eds) *Living with Chronic Illness: the experience of patients and their families*, London: Unwin Hyman.

Pollock, K. (1988) 'On the nature of social stress: production of a modern mythology', *Social Science and Medicine* 26: 381–92.

Radley, A. (1984) 'The embodiment of social relations in coronary heart disease', *Social Science and Medicine* 19: 1227–34.

Radley, A. (1988) *Prospects of Heart Surgery: psychological adjustment to coronary bypass grafting*, New York: Springer-Verlag.

Radley, A. (1989) 'Style, discourse and constraint in adjustment to chronic illness', *Sociology of Health and Illness* 11: 230–52.

Robinson, I. (1990) 'Personal narratives, social careers and medical courses: analysing life trajectories in autobiographies of people with multiple sclerosis', *Social Science and Medicine* 30: 1173–86.

Rogers, W.S. (1991) *Explaining Health and Illness: an exploration of diversity*, London: Harvester Wheatsheaf.

Romanyshyn, R.D. (1982) *Psychological Life: From Science to Metaphor*, Milton Keynes: Open University Press.

Roth, J.A. and Conrad, P. (eds) (1987) *Research in the Sociology of Health Care, vol. 6*, The Experience and Management of Chronic Illness, Greenwich, Connecticut: JAI Press Inc.

Sacks, O. (1982) *Awakenings* (rev. edn), London: Pan Books.

Scheper-Hughes, N. and Lock, M.M. (1986) 'Speaking "truth" to illness: metaphors, reification, and a pedagogy for patients', *Medical Anthropology Quarterly* 17: 137–40.

Sontag, S. (1979) *Illness as Metaphor*, London: Allen Lane.

Strauss, A. (1975) *Chronic Illness and the Quality of Life*, Saint Louis: Mosby.

Taussig, M.T. (1980) 'Reification and the consciousness of the patient', *Social Science and Medicine* 14B: 3–13.

Voysey, M. (1975) *A Constant Burden: the reconstitution of family life*, London: Routledge & Kegan Paul.

Wilden, A. (1972) *System and Structure: essays in communication and exchange*, London: Tavistock Publications.

Williams, G. (1984) 'The genesis of chronic illness: narrative reconstruction', *Sociology of Health and Illness* 6: 174–200.

7 Why do the victims blame themselves?

Mildred Blaxter

This investigation of what it means to say that 'the victims blame themselves' is presented as an example of the interaction of qualitative and quantitative methods. The question, raised by the inevitably superficial results of larger-scale surveys, is: Why do those who are most vulnerable to the environment seem to be most likely to stress self-blame for illness and self-responsibility for health? Can a biographical approach suggest some answers?

There are, of course, two perspectives on the determinants of illness, and especially the causes of social inequality in health: the idea that illhealth is primarily 'self-inflicted', and has behavioural causes, and the view that the major causes are structural and located in the environment. The extent to which people themselves subscribe to one view or the other is a topic which surveys often investigate, and though the alternatives are not necessarily mutually exclusive, the brief questions of surveys ('What is the cause of heart disease?', 'Do you think people are responsible for their own illnesses?'), perhaps with forced-choice answers, tend to create dichotomies. One consistent finding is that although most people, of whatever social group, have learned very well the self-responsible lessons of health promotion, it is those who are most 'unequal' and most exposed to environmental risk who are least likely also to be aware of the structural perspective. Those who are in the lowest social classes, or have the least education, are most likely to confine their explanations to behavioural causes. The idea that the socially fortunate may be healthier is often flatly resisted.

THE SURVEY EVIDENCE

As evidence of this, a brief summary is offered of data deriving from the Health and Lifestyle Survey (Cox *et al.*, 1987; Blaxter 1990), a national sample survey, conducted by interviewers, of just over 9,000 respondents of all ages 18 and over. The design and analysis of the sections on beliefs and attitudes of this particular survey were strongly influenced by the experience of qualitative work. The relevant questions – about the causes of specific diseases, about the healthiness of the respondent's life and the perception of 'healthy' behaviour, about effects on health 'nowadays' for society in general, about the reasons for naming a 'healthy other person', and about attitudes to various health-related areas of life – were, deliberately, asked several times, in different contexts and in different ways, and almost always in open-ended format. Thus, the conclusions which follow are derived from the patterns of reply to many different questions throughout the survey schedule.

This method permitted the analysis to accommodate, in an imitation of qualitative methods, the sometimes contradictory and seemingly confused answers which any individual can produce on the complex subject of health. In particular, context was shown to be all-important. When the questions were about specific, named diseases, behavioural answers were overwhelmingly predominent: poor diet or lack of exercise could be the cause of almost any chronic disease. For illhealth in the abstract, considering 'what makes people unhealthy', voluntary behaviours were again primarily indicted, with little differentiation by social class or education. A surprising number of people asserted that more people smoked nowadays, compared with a generation ago, and illegal drugs received a perhaps undue emphasis. In the context of their own health and their own lives, rather fewer gave behavioural replies, as common sense might suggest: nevertheless, this was still the most popular form of answer: my life is unhealthy because I can't control my weight, because I smoke; it is healthy because I take exercise, because I watch my diet.

Some of the survey questions were designed to elicit descriptions of the nature of health, rather than the causes of illness. Even in these, it was notable that a minority of people could define health only in terms of behaviour: the simulacrum, in Crawford's (1984) terms, has become the thing itself. A quite typical reply to 'Why do you call [a chosen person] healthy?' was 'I call her healthy because she goes jogging and she doesn't drink alcohol'. The extreme view that a virtuous life was synonymous with health was expressed by one lady who said 'Why do I call her healthy? Well, she leads a proper respectable life, so of course she's never ill'.

The alternative view, that structural or economic factors such as prosperity or poverty, enforced ways of living, or the external environment, were crucial for health, was mentioned additionally and quite frequently for society at large, very infrequently as an influence on one's own health or illness, and barely at all as a cause of specific disease. This contextual difference might be expected. It was notable, however, that whether the context was society or self, or whether one was talking of the bad effects of poverty and the inner city or the good effects of prosperity and an unpolluted environment, these factors were more likely to be mentioned by the rich than the poor, and by those in non-manual occupations rather than those who did manual work.

Similarly, work as a good influence on their own health was mentioned more commonly by men in semi-or unskilled occupations – usually on the grounds of exercise, or an outdoor life – than those in professional or managerial jobs. Among semi/unskilled workers, 13 per cent said that their work kept them healthy, compared with 9 per cent of skilled workers and 4 per cent of professionals. Work-related factors as unhealthy in their own lives – because of stress, overwork, working conditions, or unemployment – were cited by 6 per cent of professional and managerial men, and less than 1 per cent of unskilled workers.

It can be concluded, on the evidence of this one large-scale survey at least, that the lessons of public policy and health education – 'you are responsible for your health' – have been accepted, or at least that the population is aware of the 'correct' answers to give about the causes of health and illhealth. And, though it depends on the context in which the question is asked, it is those with higher incomes or better education who are also likely to be aware of the evidence of sociology and social epidemiology which stresses structural and environmental factors.

It must be asked, of course, whether these findings are general. In the influential work of Pill and Stott (1985a, 1985b, 1986) working-class mothers were described as having an amoral concept of causality, primarily wedded to a germ theory; nevertheless in reply to the generalized question 'I wonder what you yourself thought were the main reasons for people being ill?' the most popular category of reply apart from 'germs' related to lifestyle factors. These comprised 40 per cent of the answers, with only 15 per cent assigned to the category of environmental. A more superficial but general-population study (Blaxter 1985), in which people were asked what was unhealthy about their own lives, found that 83 per cent stressed behavioural factors, and that these were the only answers likely to be offered by those with lower income or less education.

The direct questions: 'Do you think that there are differences in the health of office workers compared with manual workers? The rich compared with the poor? The employed compared with the unemployed?' were asked of his respondents by Calnan (1987). The sample here was small, but the results clear: higher social classes were more likely to agree that the health of the rich was better, and to agree that unemployment was bad for health. Almost half the social class IV or V sample refused to believe that the unskilled had, in general, poorer health than professionals. A typical explanation, from one working-class respondent, was:

> 'Well, I think those in an office, they get bad backs ... those that work in a factory all day are working hard. I mean, they're healthier than lazing about in an office.'
>
> (Calnan 1987: 75)

It thus appears that the data of the Health and Lifestyle Survey is, indeed, supported by the findings of smaller studies.

THE SEARCH FOR EXPLANATIONS

Why should this be so? There are possible explanations of a rather facile nature. It could be argued, for instance, that although this emphasis on the behavioural, as a taught response, has been generally very well learned, alternative or additional modes of explanation are more available to those who are better educated or more exposed to 'scientific' media presentations. The middle class are also more likely to belong to contemporary consumerist and environmentalist movements. It might also be suggested that these findings are no more than an artefact of method: the more articulate are more likely to give elaborate answers in the survey situation, and the less well educated or those without a ready vocabulary of abstract concepts are likely to seek the line of least resistance and give the easiest answers perceived to be the approved ones. Certainly, it was true in the Health and Lifestyle Survey that education of the respondent was, in general, clearly associated with the length of their open-ended replies or the number of different concepts that an individual expressed.

Are such explanations sufficient? If they are given time to express themselves in a situation less reminiscent of a 'test', is it true that those who are in the poorest social and economic circumstances are still least likely to place the blame for illhealth on their environment? And if it is, how do the disadvantaged, in fact, interpret the relationship between their health and the circumstances of their lives? To answer these questions, ideally, new and clearly focused research should be mounted. In the absence of this ideal, there is the possibility of an alternative strategy: to return to a re-analysis of the qualitative material which initially provided some of the themes guiding the analysis of the Health and Lifestyle Survey.

THE QUALITATIVE DATA

The data referred to are long tape-recorded conversations with a group of 47 Scottish women of about 50 years old (Blaxter and Paterson 1982). For other purposes of the study, they had been randomly selected from women who, at the time of their first childbearing 30 or so years before, were in social classes IV or V, and whose adult daughters lived in the same city and were still in the lowest social classes. Thus they belonged to families, neither geographically nor socially mobile, who were likely to have some generations of economic deprivation behind them: a group among whom the relationship between social circumstances and ideas about the cause of illhealth could be clearly tested. The data used here consist of interviews, usually lasting for an hour and often much longer, in which the conversation was guided to cover the woman's health and health history, and her attitudes to illness, doctors and health services.

It must first be noted that the personal and family histories of the women demonstrated not only social deprivation in past generations, in their own childhoods, and at the time of their childbearing (in the early 1950s), but also the very clear association of this deprivation with illhealth. As Herzlich and Pierret (1984) noted of their French respondents, 'the memory of the terrors of the past remained astonishingly vivid'. Diphtheria and scarlet fever had swept through families:

> 'Because I remember when I was taken away with scarlet fever. I mean, that night is as clear to me as though it happened last week. I wis only four, right enough, but I remember the hospital being packed wi' kids. My husband – there was him and his two brothers – the three of them were taken out o' the house one night and my husband wasnae expected to come back. And after he did come back from the hospital he took it again.'
>
> (G37)

Six of the 47 women had had TB, and several of their own children: one woman described how her son had caught TB from 'sharing a bed with a lodger, when he came home from sea – we didn't know he had it, you see'. A stark lack of adequate food, clothing and housing was described in the days before the Second World War:

> 'I always had sore throats, septic throats and that. Before I had diphtheria we stayed in an old house – my mother blamed that. We'd only one room and there was six o' us in one room, two beds in one room at that time. An' your sink was just on the stair an' outside was your toilet.'
>
> (G3)

As young women in the 1950s their circumstances had been little better. Many husbands had been working away from home or otherwise absent, and almost all the women began married life either subletting crowded rooms from parents or other relatives, or renting crowded, damp slum property often without running water or inside sanitation. They represented themselves, at that time, as having little control over their fertility. Over half had conceived their first child before marriage, and twenty-nine of the forty-seven women had borne four or more children.

They were very conscious that part of the illhealth of the past had been due to an absence of medical services, and told many stories of not being able to afford or obtain care:

> 'When you had to pay for a doctor – well, to this day my mother still says that wa the reason I took rheumatic fever. Cos I took scarlet fever – and I was ill for a few days, and my mother took me to the dispensary. Now, I had to walk there, cos my mother didn't have the tramcar fare. With the result – I got my chill – we had to walk to the dispensary because it was free there, we couldn't afford to pull in a doctor. Cos my mother would have had the doctor in her house – well, at least twice a week, because she had eight of us.'
>
> (G1)

> 'My father had a duodenal ulcer and a gastric ulcer. Now, when we was little – she had eight, nine kids, twins twice – she got a shillin' to keep twins aff the National Assistance Board cos my father was an invalid ... at that time you got fit [what] you cried [called] Parish. Now if you was ill, you didnae pay for your operations but you didnae get your Parish. So therefore your wife and kids did without. So therefore my father had to bide and chop these sticks to keep his kids fed and dee without his operation. Now, when he did get his operation the cancer had been there that long – 25 years in agony.'
>
> (G12)

They were, however, very conscious that 'things had changed'. These family stories were usually told in the context of praise for the National Health Service, universally given credit (together with the 'medical advances' that had provided a cure for TB and, in their eyes, had been responsible for 'conquering' the childhood killers of the past) for major advances in health. G12, above, concluded by saying 'We hinna got that worry nowadays'.

Many of the women were of rural background. This acknowledgement of the effects of poverty produced some conflict with another strong and almost universal theme: the wish to present the days of their youth as in some sense 'healthier', with simple good food, fresh air and sensible living. This was an obvious appeal to a 'golden age' of the past, a response to all they disliked about modern life or all that irritated them about the way in which their grandchildren were brought up; in part, it represented the childhood memories of the rural as opposed to the urban, perhaps typical of a generation experiencing the period of rural depopulation. One woman described a tragic childhood:

> 'My mother had ten altogether – six of us survived. She died in the April and I was 13 in the May. That's when we lost her ... I kept the family together, on my own, going to school as well. And then I left school at 14 and went out to work on the farms.'
>
> (G30)

and later in the interview described at length all the chronic illnesses and early deaths of her siblings. She herself – though by definition the survivor – suffered from chronic asthma. Nevertheless, when the conversation turned to general influences on health and illness, she had strongly held views:

> 'We were a healthy family. The country people are more healthy than the town people. They have more fresh air, there's not so much traffic, factories, things like that. And we lived off the land, more or less, there wasn't so much tinned stuff and things like that... . Their whole way of life has a lot to do wi' it. You're up early in the morning, your work's not finished until maybe late at night, plenty o' fresh air.'

Another example of many similar accounts was the woman who said:

> 'My father didnae work frae during the first war – he was hurt in the war, so my mother had to bring up eight of us – it wis just a case o' us getting – we got wur soup, we didnae get the best o' everything, we just got the cheapest o' everything, but it wis a' *good*. I suppose that would give us a' the chance o' better health.'
>
> (G15)

At the same time, it would certainly be untrue to say that these women did not have a clear perception of the causes of their own specific, current chronic conditions lying in past circumstances. They seemed to be saying that their simple, healthy childhoods (leaving aside infectious disease, which was simply an ever-present but unavoidable danger, now removed by medical science) had provided them with a reserve of good health, better to withstand the attacks that later life circumstances might make. At the most difficult period of their lives, which most saw as their young married days, neglect of their own health had been inevitable. One woman was clear, for instance, about the cause of her long-term arthritis:

> 'Well, put it like this, when you've got young family you've got a lot of hard work. More so when you have five. It's nae easy work. And we'd

nae washing machines, nae hot water, nae sink – well, we had a cold sink in the corner ... there was a lot of hard work, there was stone floors.'

(G19)

Another had similar views about arthritis in her knees:

> 'Gaun aboot wi' auld shoes on – gaun aboot getting my feet soakin' – maybe, if I'd taken mair care o' mysel' earlier on. But wi' kids, no money for yoursel', you couldnae dae it.'
>
> (G23)

Later, however, this same woman talked at length of the simple, austere upbringing of her own children, and explained how 'healthy' their childhoods had been by the same sort of reasoning that other women applied to their own childhoods:

> 'Well, my four was healthy. They was never pampered and wrapped up. They niver wore scarfs and hats in the winter time. They were jist out in a' weathers. And they jist ate a' thing that was going. And yet they were healthy.'

To neglect their own health in the way they now admitted they had done meant that they were responsible, but on the other hand no one could have behaved differently:

> 'Three times in the city hospital with tuberculosis – I called it neglect. Well, I had pleurisy before my twins were born, and I cracked my ribs just before A. was born, and I had pleurisy, and I had naebody in, wi' six o' them, you know. And I had pleurisy, and there was naebody to look efter me, I just used to come an' get my poultice and heat it at the fire and put it back on. It was really neglect – my own – well, no my own fault, I had to look efter my bairns, you understand.'
>
> (G7)

Many other women similarly struggled to reconcile a strong sense of self-responsibility with the conviction that all their health problems stemmed from childbearing and the difficult days of early motherhood. To present the process as one of self-sacrifice and 'good' motherhood was an obvious solution:

> 'When they were young, if I was ill, I couldn't afford to be ill and that was all there was to it. Because he was at sea and there was naebody. There wasn't anyone to watch the kids. If I was ill I still had to get up and work, you know – you couldn't be ill.'
>
> (G25)

IMMEDIATE CAUSES

This was all in the past, and things were different now. All the women felt themselves to be in at least 'comfortable' circumstances now. The privations of the 1950s were the bad old days, and now the NHS was available. In discussing their more recent illness, or the day-to-day fluctuations in their chronic conditions, the self-responsibility theme was paramount. A few complaints were ascribed to the environment, usually the weather or the immediate environment of their housing: 'dampness in these houses', 'the bedroom walls are running', 'there's something in this water'. Generally, these seemed to be expressions of dissatisfaction with their present house, in situations where they wanted to move and had perhaps got a 'doctor's line' in support of their application for different council housing. The women did not belong to more middle-class pure air or unadulterated food lobbies, and to complain about more general 'dangers of modern life' would have gone against their firm knowledge or conviction that living circumstances had improved. Nor did they perceive any dangers in over-medicalization, in any real way: many described how they 'didn't like pills' or criticized those who relied on them, but in fact they were observed to be very heavy users of prescriptions from their doctors. There were perhaps two exceptions to this trust of prescribed drugs: the contraceptive pill, and psychotropics. Both of these could be the cause of many problems. They were special, it seemed, because so intimately connected with the life events – marriage, childbearing, tragedies, growing older – which were the framework of their medical biographies.

Their working history – on the farms, or the cold, unpleasant work of fish processing when they were young, the hard work of hospitals, shops, and domestic service in later life – also represented both the hardships of their lives, and their strength in endurance. Work was also an important part of biography, and could be associated with the beginning of a variety of illnesses.

At a more superficial level, however, it was behavioural causes that were offered for almost every disease – certainly in the abstract, or in other people, but also for oneself. This seemed largely to be the recital of what they had been taught. Twenty-three of the forty-seven women suffered from chronic chest complaints, of this group twenty smoked, and all except one volunteered their smoking as a cause or at least a contributory factor. Lengthy reports were given of their interactions with doctors on the topic, in the course of which the women might express some degree of scepticism: 'If I did stop smoking I'd die of a heart attack overweight' 'I've smoked since I was 14, so if there's anything going to happen it'll happen'. Nevertheless, at later points in the interview the association of smoking with bronchitis would always, and repeatedly, be ruefully acknowledged: 'that's smoking, of course', 'I'm breathless, I have to put it down to smoking'. Similar friction with doctors, spirited self-defences, but on the whole guilty agreement that it was their own fault, related to obesity. 'Blood pressure' was often the sufferer's own fault, for 'rushing around' or 'doing too much' and several other disease conditions were subject to discussion about 'what one had done' to get them: diabetes was described by more than one woman, for instance, as being caused by an over-fondness for sugar.

HEALTH AS BIOGRAPHY

It thus seems that, if the women are considered as a group in this way, survey results are supported. Behaviour was the simplest 'public' answer to 'what is the cause of illness', the known 'expected' answer, and the one which they believed was medically authorized (Cornwell 1984). To consider typical answers in this way, however, is largely to misrepresent the women's real thinking about cause. If, in a different manner of analysis, a single respondent's way of thinking is traced back and forwards throughout the hour or two of conversation, these answers are seen in context. In fact, nothing has one cause. Alternatives are tried out, rejected, associated with each other, traced from one period of life to another. Examples are given of different cases, and the different factors that might apply are reasoned out. An attempt is made to achieve that 'experiential coherence' (as distinct from abstract, theoretical coherence) which has been shown (e.g. Pinder 1992) to be sought by those trying to interpret their own chronic disease.

Obviously, this is less easy to illustrate briefly. However, three examples follow, confined to the single story of the woman's own current and most salient health problems, which illustrate some typical themes. In these stories, as Cornwell also found, causal theories move between internal and external factors: 'the illness was not portrayed as something that could be separated from the person or the circumstances of their personal biography' (1984: 161). The women seek to answer the 'Why me? Why now?' questions in a way which, in Herzlich and Pierret's (1984) words, 'transcends the search for causes and becomes a quest for meaning'.

G14 – aged 54, 12 children

The main complaint chronic bronchitis: began with 'change of life at the time'. But also	life stage
began when husband, 'a war pensioner', could not work and she 'took on a really old house' with the idea of lodgers. 'And then I took ill. I had a' the work	stress, social circumstances

and a' thing, you see.'	
The bronchitis 'started off with flu, and developed from that.'	
Doctors told her it was smoking, and 'I stopped for nine months!' (But claims was better when she started again.)	(?) behaviour
Second, later, account of beginning of bronchitis: had a bout of pneumonia and neglected it, because she will never 'give in' to illness. 'Cos that was me, wi' pneumonia and bronchitis, walking down to the City hospital' (very long account of resisting hospitalization, on this and other occasions)	self-neglect
'I said, I'm nae gaun intae nae bed, I've a' these bairns at hame, I'm gaun back.' 'It's got to beat me first afore I'll call the doctor.'	life stage 'not giving in'
At about the same time she had a bad fall on ice in the street, 'Something gaed intae my leg' Secondary trouble is still pains in the leg and arms. 'It wis after that I first got the cold, and it went to my chest.'	effects of trauma
At present has laryngitis, but 'I'm blaming the weather.' 'And smoking disnae help.'	weather behaviour
The continued pain is perhaps 'just wear and tear on the spine'. Of course 'You couldnae expect onything else, wi' all that bairns.' She had two children after 40, which was 'too auld, maybe.'	natural ageing childbearing
Also has 'a kinda knot at the back o' my neck', which may be affecting the spine, but 'I think it's just a cyst maybe'.	
Also suffers from migraine. Considers whether it is perhaps associated with her neck? But 'I've had migraine since the last one was born.'	childbearing
Nevertheless describes self as healthy. 'The only recipe I say is nae to lie down wi' the least little thing that's wrang wi' ye. Sometimes, if ye ging awa' and do a little bit of washing or something, you forget a' aboot your pains.'	self-responsibility 'not giving in'

G40 – aged 53, three children

'Healthwise OK' but does suffer from bothersome pains in the hand and arms. Probably 'just rheumatics ... at	natural ageing

my time o' life'.	
Had feared heart trouble, but since the doctor 'just gave painkillers' this was evidence that there 'was nothing else showing'.	
Later, says was also told 'disc is worn in the spine'.	(?) ageing
Rejects an explanation in terms of 'just ageing'; suggests it could be due to being 'hurt doing acrobatics as a child'. 'It's a permanent injury in my neck.'	effect of trauma
Subsequently, almost casually mentions surgery which had involved 'taking lumps out of my breast and under my arms'. This was after she had her children, and 'they did say to me it was shifting intae the new home, wi' stone floors, and being in the scullery, and the steel frame windows, and the dampness must have gone right up through me.'	childbearing physical environment
Theme of heart disease recurs several times. Long discussion of how her mother, and a nephew, and 'a' my sisters has died wi' heart attacks.'	heredity
Returns to own pains. 'When I had this pain I thought, "O my God .... ."' Should perhaps take more care.	
self-responsibility	
'They say work never kills you. You know how it is – well. I go on and on – I mean, I should sit a lot more than I do ... [but] I dinna think I would be happy that way.'	overwork
Discussion of what promotes health generally: 'I think its just wi' theirsels really'. Overeating has a great deal to do with illness, 'A glutton is the worst person there is'. 'But I'm an afa' devil for sugar, mind.'	behaviour
Expands later on self-responsibility for health, although heart attacks have to be excepted – 'There's nae really no warning or nothing... I mean, just like you dinna ken when your motor's going to break down. It's just the same thing.'.	some diseases unpredictable

G19 – aged 43, five children

Major current problem is that she is waiting for a hysterectomy, 'I'm aye awfu' tired'. Ever since the fifth child (at 30) 'I've felt really tired and done.'	childbearing

Has also had bronchitis all her life. It 'comes back wi' the weather'. 'And of course I smoke.' It started with 'teething bronchitis' and runs through the family: 'My father had it, and my sister and myself, had it, and my daughter has it aff me, and her baby here, seven weeks old and it already has a whistle, so it must be taking it aff the mother.'	weather behaviour heredity
Returns to gynaecological problems. 'It's mental strain – and bringing up five kids is bound to leave something, I mean it's a' right for him [husband] – he gaed round the world when my kids was little, he cam home and put me pregnant and gaed awa' again!'	stress
Further talk of family history of chest problems, which leads to story of own mother's death from cancer.	heredity
Gynaecological problems: the state she is in is largely 'my ain fault' for not consulting earlier. 'It's jist anither phase of life. There's different things in life occurs, and you go on to anither phase of life. Me, I've come through all I've come through, it's only me I'm hurting now' (by neglect of health).	self-neglect life stage
Nevertheless 'healthy enough'. No reason to coddle self now. In comparison with days when children were young, life is easy. At that time she was almost overwhelmed with illness, but pulled herself through by her own efforts.	stress social circumstances
Returns to talk about mother. 'This is aye at the back o' my mind. Naebody kens until you're actually opened.'	some diseases unpredictable
Seems to retreat to talk again of bronchitis, which is more familiar and understandable: 'I mean, we're all made of an impression on our ancestors, arn't we? So if you've a weakness it must come out some way.'	heredity

These summaries are necessarily devoid of the small details which give them life. One extended quotation is added from the last respondent above, as an example of the lively, sophisticated and independent way in which the theme of stress and resentment as the cause of illness could be worked out. It also shows how, as Crawford (1984) noted, 'in the mind-over-matter formulation, one discipline is substituted for another': illness again becomes the sufferer's fault.

'When I wis bringin' up my kids, I was forever in at the doctor and I had like a chemist shop – I had tablets to mak' me sleep, I had tablets for heidaches, an' tablets for stomach aches, an' I just said tae mysel' tablets, tablets – I ta'en them a' an' I pit them in the bucket. I says, now they're nae helpin' me, I've got tae dae it mysel. So I got to work an' worked things oot mysel'.... When I first got that heidaches, I thought I was goin' aff the heid. They put me to the [psychiatric hospital]. He [husband] says, "You're a nut". I says, "Well, I'll be a nut, but I'll find out I am a nut, I'll ging to a psychiatrist." A' they asked about was sex – well, it had nuthin' a'dee wi' sex. An' then it dawned on me fit it wis – the strain o' the kids were gettin' ower much for me an' I wis against him [husband] for aye bein' awa'! See? An' then, when things would crack up, I'd maybe smack them, for maybe little. I would sit doon an' greet – I shouldn't have hutten them. Ken? An' the heidaches would get worse an' worse – an' worse ... . Ken, gettin' tae ken things, has a lot to dee wi' it – ignorance is a lot tae dee wi' bad health.'

(G19)

CHAINS OF CAUSE

Several themes run throughout these accounts. First, there is the constant emphasis on life events, especially those identified with their female roles: childbearing, the care of elderly parents and their deaths, the menopause, widowhood, the deaths of children. Almost every chronic condition had its 'real' origins in one of these events. In particular, childbearing had been the crucial event: 'a woman's never the same after she's had children' was a popular aphorism.

These were all links in the chain of cause. A second notable feature of the accounts was the strain to connect, to present a health history as a chain of cause and effect, with each new problem arising from previous ones. There was a common concept of one disease 'going into' another, and many causes were sought in past injuries. A cough would 'go into' bronchitis, meningitis was caused by 'a knock', accidents many years before were blamed for arthritis. Accidents, like surgery, were assaults upon the body, unnatural breakings or openings which would leave it susceptible. Occasionally, disease might be seen as striking randomly: cancer is the most common example, though it must be noted that the reluctance to discuss cancer at length seemed also to be an expression of a taboo. Often the disease was not directly named, or the voice was dropped to a whisper. For most diseases, however, cause was not random. The women resisted the idea that one part of their body might have 'gone wrong' at one time, and another at another, without there being any connection. One thing must lead to another: there must be a logical biography.

These chains of cause stretched back through generations. Thus heredity and familial patterns were another pervasive theme in the talk of their own disease. In part, this was simply a natural human tendency towards 'pattern making', and, since families in the past had been large and certain diseases very prevalent, there was a high likelihood that if patterns were sought they could be found. Family weaknesses often lay in stomachs, or chests, or some other part of the body: 'They've all been bothered with their legs'. Alternatively, families could have some inherent strengths, resilience to certain types of condition. These discussions of family history, often very long, were commonly quite sophisticated, with the women working out in great detail exact degrees of relationship, the evidence of changes in environment (many older members of families had emigrated), or the different likelihoods of infection, direct inheritance, or 'susceptibility'. G37, for instance, explained:

> 'I think family traits have a habit o' – you know, cropping up. You might have a family that's prone to rheumatics. Rheumatics aren't infectious, but if it runs in a family, to me, you know, as it comes down the line, there's always going to be somebody that's sorta inclined to take that. In this climate... .'

This was set in the context of a recital of the lives and deaths of her own parents, siblings, and grandparents, and then of her husband's family. A digression considered the effects of voluntary lifestyles: her paternal grandfather died young, but he was a well-known drinker; on the other hand so did his father, 'and he was a very religious churchgoing man, he didn't smoke or drink'. The conclusion was:

> '... families can be long-living families or short-living families. I think it must be something to do with the genes.'

This fondness for familial 'explanations', as for connecting up the events of their lives, could be understood as a liking for continuity, a desire to give meaning to their lives. Their family histories, together with their own experiences, constituted their identity. Their present health status, including all the emerging problems of middle-age, had to be accommodated into that identity.

HEALTH AS MORAL IDENTITY

In particular, they wished to present a moral identity. Moral opprobrium attached, not to *having* illnesses, but in 'lying down' to them. A woman who complained, who made a fuss, who allowed illhealth to interfere with her duties, was a 'poor thing', to be pitied or scorned. Almost without exception, they themselves were presented as models of stoicism:

> 'I never lie down to illness – I've gotten up in the morning wi' a migraine and gone to work. Nearly killed me, mind, but I've gone ... I'd rather be out in the company, you know, an' you're busy. I mean, if you're in the house you've still to make a meal and light the fire – you just canna lie. Well, I canna, I canna lie if I know the fire wants cleaning, no matter how bad I am. I've never been off work, never. You get some that stops off with the least thing ... .'
>
> (G22)

They were firm adherents to the Protestant ethic. Hard work was virtue, virtue was rewarded, and health must be the reward of industry. So almost all were quick to describe themselves as 'healthy', no matter how long the list of illnesses they then went on to describe. This applied to their family members as well, even though they may have had many chronic diseases and died at an early age:

> 'My mother was aye healthy – she wis up at 5 o'clock in the morning, she had a' her work done, she wis oot in the toon half-past 8, she had a' her shopping done. She was real healthy, like.'
>
> (G7)

These attitudes may obviously be characteristic of the particular culture of NE Scotland. But perhaps it is also an example of one of the paradoxes of 'embodiment' noted by Turner (1984): that, while the whole Christian tradition of the West affirms that the body is but weak flesh, the location of sin, it is also 'an instructive site of moral purpose and intentions', with health as the sign of moral well-being.

IDENTITY CREATED THROUGH INTERACTION

People do not, of course, create their biographies and their identities in a vacuum. It is obvious that the process not only takes place within a cultural context, but is also a continual interaction with others, especially parents, spouses, other family and neighbours. Although the data here were, ideally, collected in one-to-one private conversations between interviewer and subject, some evidence about this process did emerge. In crowded and gregarious households privacy was not always possible, and there are a few interviews where other family members – usually husbands or daughters – were present, at least for part of the time. It seems of interest to ask whether these presentations of self were – in a situation where they were being offered to a relative stranger – likely to be challenged, or likely to be reinforced.

Within the family, there were in fact frequent examples of support, and none of challenge. That this was how the woman *was* was a well-known fact.

A few of the husbands who happended to hear part of the interview expressed some cynicism about 'all this women's talk', and provided a chorus of comment, sometimes with friendly bickering and sometimes with an undercurrent of spite, but never with any serious challenge to the woman's image as someone who would not 'give in' to illness. Moreover, several women (not in the presence of their husbands) suggested that these stoical attitudes were the direct result of being placed in women's roles, in a culture where men had expected their wives to serve them, and where men's household comfort and working capacity took priority. Men 'who has pampered their wives' were not spoken of with any particular favour: they did their wives no service. The women's daughters did not necessarily agree: times had changed. Nevertheless they, too, supported and amplified the 'strength through adversity' theme of their mothers' biographies, using as their evidence the often-heard stories of their childhoods.

These fortuitous occasions where family interactions were observed cannot necessarily be regarded as representative data. The joint creation of biographies within families is a topic deserving research in its own right. There did, however, seem to be glimpses here of the processes by which biographies evolve and are reinforced.

IDENTITY AND DEPRIVATION

This intensely moral view of health meant, of course, that – even while they were recounting all the health deprivations of the past – the women were as reluctant to describe their families as unhealthy as they were to label themselves. If actually challenged, they would reject ideas about class inequalities, echoing the respondents of Calnan quoted earlier:

> 'I dinna think their surroundings has onything to dee wi' it. I mean, you could have ony God's amount o' money and the best o' everything, and you could have the unhealthiest child in the world. An' you could hae nothing, and hae to work and bring them up yoursel', an' you'll find you've got the healthiest kids.'
>
> (G40)

They were aware, as they offered their biographies, that they had little to boast of in terms of material success. They could, however, be proud of their large, close families and of the virtues – simplicity of lifestyle, hard work, triumph over adversity – which they saw as pre-eminent. Those in richer circumstances probably lacked these virtues, and could not be rewarded with better health.

CONCLUSION

In summary, it seems probable that if these women had been asked the brief direct questions of the Health and Lifestyle Survey, their answers would have been in accordance with the class patterns found. Illness was primarily one's own responsibility, not only at the superficial level of quickly-offered survey responses, but also at a deeper level of claiming responsibility for one's own identity. They did not dwell on class inequalities because, though they were very conscious of the perils of the environment in the past, by contrast life seemed to be largely without such dangers now. They were perfectly capable of holding in equilibrium ideas which might seem opposed: the ultimate cause, in the story of the deprived past, of their current illhealth, but at the same time their own responsibility for 'who they were'; the inevitability of illhealth, given their biographies, but at the same time guilt if they were forced to 'give in' to illness. With this emphasis on selfhood and self-responsibility, and their knowledge of greatly improved general social circumstances, a rejection of ideas about (contemporary) 'inequality' was understandable.

Many such qualitative studies have shown that people reconstruct biomedical concepts, including those of aetiology, in the light of their own biographies. Perhaps sociologists and social epidemiologists may have to accept that their concepts, too, may have little reality at the level of individual perceptions.

REFERENCES

Blaxter, M. (1985) 'Self-definition of health status and consulting rates in primary care', *Quarterly Journal of Social Affairs*, 1, 133–71.

Blaxter, M. (1990) *Health and Lifestyles*, London: Routledge.

Blaxter, M. and Paterson, E. (1982) *Mothers and Daughters*, London: Heinemann.

Calnan, M. (1987) *Health and Illness: the lay perspective*, London: Tavistock Publications.

Cornwell, J. (1984) *Hard-earned Lives: Accounts of Health and Illness from East London*, London: Tavistock Publications.

Cox, B.D., Blaxter, M. *et al.* (1987) *The Health and Lifestyle Survey. Preliminary Report*, London: Health Promotion Research Trust.

Crawford, R. (1984) 'A cultural account of "health": control, release and the social body', in J.B. McKinlay (ed.) *Issues in the Political Economy of Health Care*, London: Tavistock Publications.

Herzlich, C., and Pierret, J. (1984) *Illness and Self in Society*, Baltimore: Johns Hopkins University Press.

Pill, R. and Stott, N.C. (1985a) 'Prevention procedures and practices among working-class women: new data and fresh insights', *Social Science and Medicine* 21: 975–83.

Pill, R. and Stott, N.C. (1985b) 'Choice or chance: further evidence on ideas of illness and responsibility for health', *Social Science and Medicine* 20: 981–91.

Pill, R. and Stott, N.C. (1986) 'Looking after themselves: health protective behaviour among British working-class women', *Health Education Research* 1: 111–19.

Pinder, R. (1992) 'Coherence and incoherence: doctors' and patients' perspectives on the diagnosis of Parkinson's Disease', *Sociology of Health and Illness* 14: 1.

Turner, B.S. (1984) *The Body and Society*, Oxford: Blackwell.

8 Towards the reconstruction of an organic mental disorder

Tom Kitwood

The argument of this chapter is as follows. Senile dementia has been constructed by a cluster of discourses, of which the dominant one is grounded in medical science. This discourse, however, is far less coherent than it is commonly taken to be. Our understanding of dementia and dementia care can be reconstructed in relation to a discourse which gives central place to personhood and interpersonal relations. The creation of such a discourse challenges both material interests and psychological defences.

In the whole field of modern psychiatry, as it has developed since the founding work of Kraepelin and others around the turn of the century, senile dementia stands as one of the most puzzling of all afflictions. Superficially the primary degenerative dementias appear to be paradigmatic of the category 'organic mental disorder', and this is how they are generally presented in standard textbooks and popular accounts. In fact, however, when the details are scrutinized, almost nothing – not even the alleged organicity – is assured. The discourse generated by medical science is so dominant, and supported by such power and prestige, that its anomalies, self-contradictions and non sequiturs are obscured from view. A tremendous amount of social construction and repair work has been necessary to keep this discourse from falling into ruins.

These problematic features of senile dementia are not simply an intriguing puzzle for sociologists of knowledge. The 'regime of truth' surrounding dementia has a direct bearing on the lives of many millions of people throughout the world, as the great demographic shift towards an older population takes its course. A typical urban area in the industrialized world, with a population of 250,000, is likely to contain some 2,000 sufferers from moderate, and 1,000 from severe dementia; the great majority of these will be in the over-eighties age range (Ineichen, 1987). There is much controversy about how people who have a dementing illness should be treated medically and cared for socially. If we can grasp the nature of the discourses surrounding dementia, the understanding and actions which they both do and do not permit, the psychological defences and material interests which are involved, this may be highly liberating. The dominant discourse may, perhaps, be prized open, and new possibilities envisaged for easing this vast burden of human suffering.

THE DOMINANT DISCOURSE

By the middle part of this century the main dementing illnesses of old age were becoming well known. As compared to today they were not so salient in psychiatry, because the proportion of people in the older age range, and particularly the 'old-old', was still relatively small. It was widely believed (although without adequate supporting evidence) that the underlying cause of dementia was often the 'hardening of the arteries', and hence an insufficient supply of blood to the brain. Around this time the rest of the dementing conditions that were not associated with some clear pathology such as brain tumour were loosely grouped together as senility; it was recognized that there were various concomitant lesions in the grey matter of the cerebral cortex. Alzheimer's Disease was the name given to a relatively rare clinical entity, where a somewhat younger person (typically in his or her fifties) underwent a rather rapid dementing illness; post-mortem investigations had shown that in the brains of such persons some of the cortical tissue had degenerated drastically.

From the late 1960s, when the ageing of the population was being clearly identified as a problem, and when methods of examining brain tissue were well-developed, a number of major studies were carried out on the brains of people who had lived on into old age. These studies showed that the lesions present in the grey matter of many of those who had a dementing illness were very similar, if not identical to, those that had been identified as typical of Alzheimer's Disease. A consensus grew up that among all cases of senile dementia some 50 per cent were associated with Alzheimer-type degeneration, 10–15 per cent with failure of blood supply (due mainly to small infarcts), and 10–15 per cent with lesions of both types (Albert 1982). The remainder were accountable to tumours, infections, hormonal disorders, metabolic imbalances, hydrocephalus and other conditions.

Henceforth the largest category of senile dementias was renamed as Alzheimer's Disease. It now appeared as if the primary cause of what had previously been called senility had been identified: it was a disease process in the brain, and not ageing per se. With multi-infarct dementia the process was well understood, but for Alzheimer's Disease the underlying cause or causes were obscure. It was soon after these discoveries that Alzheimer societies began to be formed in a number of countries. The announcement of a disease entity seemed to provide an explanation, a focus for shared concern and mutual support.

As research on the brain intensified, with the aid of several new investigative techniques, dementia became more clearly demarcated from ageing per se. In some respects this must be regarded as a progressive move. It was now the clear responsibility of doctors to do all they could to make accurate differential diagnoses when a person presented symptoms of cognitive impairment. Also it became harder to dismiss a patient or a concerned relative with such platitudes as 'It's just old age'. (Evasions of this kind are, in fact, far from having disappeared, and may be expected to return in force wherever medical services are under heavy economic pressure.)

Although the 'medicalization of dementia' brought about a certain clarification it had other consequences, arguably less benign. The prime task for doctors, in dealing with those who were confused, was to ensure that all treatable causes had been identified and dealt with. This, however, accounted for only a very small proportion of all patients. The majority of the rest were consigned to the category 'primary degenerative dementia', with its two main subdivisions. In the case of Alzheimer's Disease it was (and still is) largely a matter of diagnosis by default. In the case of multi-infarction, on the other hand, some positive diagnostic evidence was available through methods of scanning. But with both types of dementia, the implication was that the condition was hopeless from the standpoint of medical science. Drugs were available, of course, for dealing with accompanying physical ailments, and there were antidepressants and tranquillizers. There was, however, no fundamental medical treatment for the brain pathology. Senility had been a vague term, blurring the distinction between those who were relatively well-preserved and those who were not. 'Primary degenerative dementia', in contrast, was presented as a clear diagnostic category, laden with doom. Its effect, it may be argued, was to exclude and stigmatize, to banish the dementia sufferer from the world of persons. Various ideas about the 'stages of dementia' were advanced, each one claiming that the end-point of a dementing illness was a state near to that of a vegetable.

From this time forward medical science, in whatever of its main branches – epidemiology, aetiology, genetics, neuropathology, pharmacology – accepted the 'organicity' of the main senile dementias as unproblematic. The core assumption, which still underpins the whole discourse, is one of simple linear causation. It may be expressed as:

X ⟶ neuropathic change ⟶ dementia

In the case of multi-infarct dementia the nature of both X and the neuropathic change are fairly well understood. General health considerations, at least, can be brought to bear in the attempt to prevent X (failure of blood supply at the capillary level) from occurring. In the case of Alzheimer's Disease there have been many advances in elucidating the neuropathology, with a growing consensus that there may, in fact, be several more-or-less distinct conditions. The identity of X remains mysterious, although many hypotheses have been put forward, and there is controversy over whether one or several causal agents are involved. Biomedical research in the field is extremely active, involving huge commitments of money by drug companies. Within this general frame, however, scientific investigation seems to be largely at an impasse.

Medical science, then, created a powerful discourse about dementia. It was 'technical' in its orientation: that is, it viewed the human being, for the purposes of research, as an extremely complex mechanism, and the problem was to discover precisely why and how the mechanism had broken down. The crucial question of how brain and mind are related was largely ignored or bypassed.

THE SUBSIDIARY DISCOURSES

Under the tutelage of the dominant discourse, and backed by such potent images as 'the death that leaves the body behind', several other discourses took form. One of these had a strongly sentimental character. It was often cast biographically, with accounts about how a person had been before, and how he or she had deteriorated as the disease took over. Frequently these accounts were accompanied by anecdotes about the dementing person's habits, both endearing and annoying, and expressions of the carer's grief. As Gubrium (1986) has shown, sometimes whole life histories were re-cast in the terms provided by the dominant discourse. The sentimental discourse was expressed also in a view of caregiving. The dementing person was taken as being, in many respects, like a child; the task was to keep that person, as far as possible, in good physical health, fed, toiletted, clean and comfortable, protected from harm. In this discourse the carer had a basic stance on the sidelines, an impotent witness to the ravages brought about by the disease, as it pursued its relentless course. Humour, courage, and an almost superhuman endurance were involved, and often religious faith was seen as playing an important part. But the task of the caregiver was assumed to be essentially hopeless.

At the professional level – in the work of nurses, careworkers, occupational therapists, clinical psychologists and others – another subsidiary discourse took form. It was that of 'behavioural management', claiming the branch of psychology that was, allegedly, the most strictly scientific as its main resource. The strongest emphasis was on things done by dementia sufferers that were troublesome for caregivers: incontinence, wandering, sleeplessness, aggression, sexual disinhibition and so on. The general aim was to re-shape behaviour into a more acceptable mould, through methods derived from operant conditioning. The resonances of behaviourism are to be found again and again in the standard care manuals, and in the talk of professionals, especially those at high level. Even Reality Orientation, which was originally conceived as a way of engaging the subjectivity of dementing persons (Folsom 1967) has often been assimilated to a behavioural discourse. In all of this there is a curious irony. The research literature shows very little evidence of constructive change that can be clearly attributable to behavioural methods per se; where success is reported, it often seems necessary to adduce explanations that include the dementia sufferer's subjectivity (Bredin 1991). The behavioural discourse serves as a kind of rhetorical adornment to care practice.

CONTRADICTIONS AND APPEARANCES

The intensive medicalization of dementia led, then, to the formation of a discourse which had a dominant and determinative place. It appeared convincing, and was backed by institutional prestige and powerful material interests. In its shadow, and not contradicting it in any serious way, there arose a number of subsidiary discourses, such as the sentimental and behavioural ones we have examined. Together, these discourses form the stock-in-trade of the standard care manuals, the stories written by family members, and the material published by the Alzheimer Societies. The lay world was presented with a bland and impenetrable facade, as if 'the truth' about dementia had been established.

Much of this, however, is illusion. In fact the dominant discourse is far from being coherent, even in its own terms. Serious anomalies and inconsistencies continue to appear; these are contained or assimilated in a way that bears a strong resemblance to the tactic of 'saving the appearances' that was adopted when the Ptolemaic system of astronomy was falling into disarray during the sixteenth century. We have already seen how the problem of brain and mind tends to be bypassed, although this must, surely, be the cornerstone of any theory in psychiatry. But there are four other areas of contradiction with which the dominant discourse cannot adequately deal (Kitwood 1990a).

The first of these has been present throughout the whole period of intensive study of brain tissue. It is that the correlation between the degree of dementia (as assessed clinically or through standard tests) and the measured extent of the damage to the grey matter is much lower than generally believed. This is true whatever neuropathological indicators are taken. In the most famous of all the studies in this area, that of Blessed, Tomlinson and Roth (1968) the correlation coefficients were in the range 0.6–0.8, which appears convincing, especially considering the relative crudity of the measures. But the authors themselves pointed out that when cases where both degree of dementia and extent of neuropathology were low, the correlations approached statistical insignificance. This was not an isolated finding. Right through to the present day postmortem investigations have produced evidence of a similar kind, whatever indices of brain damage have been used. The most serious anomalies of all arise in those cases where a person completes, apparently, the entire course of a dementing illness, going through its stages as classically described, and then the brain is found to have no neuropathic changes beyond what might be expected for one who is not cognitively impaired. These cases are known to all the major research groups in the field. (e.g. Homer *et al.* 1988).

How are these anomalies to be accounted for? One move is to point out that the methods of measurement are fairly crude, and indeed may not be sensitive to the earliest stages of neurological damage; thus the correlations would not be expected to be high. This may well be true; but if so, the assertion that dementia is caused by neuropathic change is made on the basis of faith and not of factual evidence. An alternative move is to claim that there are many problems in making a clear diagnosis; the most powerful anomalies (high dementia, low neuropathology) were in fact instances of a reversible 'pseudodementia', whose symptoms are remarkably similar to those of a true primary degenerative condition. This move 'saves the appearances' in one sense; but the cost is to undermine the validity of one of the key variables: that of 'degree of dementia', however that may be determined. Thus we reach the *pons asinorum* of dementia research. Is the ultimate criterion of dementia to be what is assessed clinically, or is it to be one or more of the various forms of neuropathology? The tendency of late has been to choose the former (McKhann *et al.* 1984). This is honest and courageous, but it leaves the anomaly unresolved.

The second major contradiction relates to aetiology. According to the dominant discourse the causes of primary degenerative dementia are entirely physical, as befits an organic mental disorder. Psychological factors such as personality or stress reactions play no part in causation. Yet the psychobiographical study of dementia is not consistent with this view. When relatives are asked to reconstruct the story of a dementing person's illness, in many cases they point to a particular event, or cluster of events, and assert it was from that time forward that the person changed, or began to go downhill. The phenomenon of 'apparent precipitation' is well known in the field of dementia care, even if not in psychiatry.

In our own research (see Kitwood 1990b), psychobiographical data were collected on forty-four persons, and in twenty-seven of these the relative pointed to one or more critical life events as precipitants. The crucial life events fall into the following categories: 1. Retirement, redundancy or major role loss; 2. Bereavement; 3. Rejection or disgrace; 4. Stressful conflict; 5. Geographical change; 6. Accident; 7. Assault or burglary; 8. Major physical illness or operation. To give one example, related to categories 1, 2 and 3; a man who had once been a professional musician had a small organ in his house, which he used to play regularly: the neighbours complained that they were being disturbed, and in a fit of pique he decided to sell it. According to his wife, on the day the organ was taken away, her husband got lost in town, and he began to dement from that time forward. In the research literature there are a few studies which point in a similar direction, such as that of Amster and Kraus (1974), who used a standard life events method.

It may be objected that it is naive to accept at face value the retrospective accounts given by family members. Perhaps a relative, in dealing with a tragic loss and all the accompanying complexities of emotion, is striving to find a pattern and a meaning, and attaches causal weight inappropriately to particular events. Or it might be claimed that some events are genuinely causal, but have directly physical explanations. For example, major surgery such as hip replacement might involve the migration of small blood clots to the brain. To write off relatives' psychological explanations as fundamentally wrong does, however, seem to be arbitrary, especially as some recent research has attested to a remarkable accuracy in carers' observations on those they are looking after (O'Connor *et al.* 1989). Moreover, it is wholly consistent with medical science to hold open the possibility that loss, change and disruption might, for some personality types, be dementogenic. Depressive reactions may be involved, and the weakening of the immune system as in other major organic disorders such as cancer. Only gross prejudice would uphold the view that there could be no psychogenic aspects in the aetiology of dementia. The burden of the proof is shifting onto those who believe there are none, to bring forward their evidence and reasons.

The third anomaly in the dominant discourse relates to a very well-known fact which simply stands on its own, unassimilated. It is that some persons who are dementing relatively slowly undergo a rapid decline in mental abilities when their life-situation is changed, or when some serious disruption occurs. Typical precipitants here are being hospitalized for assessment, being taken into respite care, or entry into a residential or nursing home. It is not uncommon for a person whose existing support system is unable to continue, and who is then taken into an institution, to deteriorate drastically, even to the point where close relatives are no longer recognized, within so short a period as three months.

These phenomena, and especially the cases where no physical trauma is involved, require explanation. Now it is possible, of course, that rapid deterioration of the kind we are concerned with here has been caused directly by an advance in brain pathology, which simply 'happened to' occur concomitantly, and then acted as a primary cause of mental decline. Such an idea is not consistent, however, with the best evidence available from neuropathology. The crucial case is Alzheimer's Disease of the early-onset type, where it is known that the pathological process is relatively rapid; but here it typically takes years rather than weeks to run its course. Also, to suppose that the deterioration is merely coincidental in every case requires a credulity that borders on superstition. It makes much more sense to suppose that 'psychological factors', in the sense of how the dementia sufferer apprehends his or her life-situation (albeit with impaired cognitions) play a key part in the course of a dementing illness.

There is yet a fourth problem for the dominant discourse. It is one which challenges it deeply, especially the idea of 'stages of dementia' which are related to the structural damage in the brain. Those who specialize in the care of dementing persons, and who are well-enough resourced to aim for excellence, repeatedly testify that some persons cease to deteriorate when their life-situation has become stable, and even undergo a degree of 'rementing', or recovery of powers that were lost (e.g. Bell and McGregor 1991). Research evidence of a systematic kind is just beginning to appear in the literature. Rovner *et al.* (1990), for example, report a comparative study of two groups of residents in institutional care. One group was given far more attention than the other, and an enriched programme of activities. After a year, the first group showed relatively little cognitive decline, whereas the second group showed the sort of decline that might typically be expected. Also, at an individual level, there are now some reports of rementing, (e.g. Roach 1985, Hope 1986). Much systematic research is needed on this important topic. Great advances would be made if it could be determined with which types of person, and with which dementing illnesses, and under what conditions, stabilization or rementing tends to occur. Even now, however, the phenomena must be acknowledged; an adequate theory of dementia must, surely, provide a place for them to be accounted for.

Anomalies such as the four discussed here can, of course, be neutralized by those who are determined to 'save the appearances' at all costs. Difficult evidence can be ignored, or explained away through what Popper called 'ad hoc modification'. It is clear, however, even now, that the main primary degenerative dementias, at the very time when they are most decisively claimed to be diseases, do not meet three of the classical criteria for calling a clinical entity a disease. There is no unique set of symptoms which clearly mark each disease off from other conditions. In no category is there a definite disease course, or set of alternative courses. And crucially, there is not a pathology which is found in every positive case, but not found in cases where the disease is not present. All the boundaries around senile dementia are, in fact, extremely vague. And, paradoxically, the entity which is most emphatically proclaimed to be a disease – Alzheimer's – is actually the least defined. The dominant discourse undoubtedly solves many practical problems, especially in providing a focus for biomedical research. What it does not do, however, is to provide the basis for a coherent explanation of the dementing process. The idea that it does so is an illusion.

'SAVING THE APPEARANCES' – ANOTHER WAY

The dominant discourse, founded as it is on medical science, clearly faces great challenges to its coherence. This will continue, so long as it takes no account of how brain and mind are related, and so long as it resolutely excludes psychological considerations at its core. Any reconstruction of theory must be such that the anomalies are dealt with better, while full place is still given to the corroborated findings of medical research.

Such reconstruction is possible. Let it be assumed that there is a basic identity between brain and mind, but a complementarity of descriptions. Thus for every mental event or state there is a corresponding functional brain event or state, 'carried' by a brain that is in a particular structural condition (Kitwood 1989). Granted this, we may look at the dementing process in terms of three categories. The first is the structural condition of the brain, arising both from the establishment of interneuronal connections and from any processes that have damaged or destroyed nerve tissue. This category is measurable in principle, although in practice it is far beyond present instrumental capability. In all persons, so the evidence suggests, the structural state of the brain is undergoing decline in the long term; there is a progressive fall-out of neurones, and pathologies of both the Alzheimer type and the infarct type are present to a small degree. The second category is hypothetical. It is the highest level of mental functioning that is possible when a person's brain is in a particular structural state. Presumably this category follows the first closely; that is, the upper limits to mental functioning are set by the structural state of the brain. The third category is the actual mental functioning of the person. Aspects of this are testable, even at the present state of the art; for example through measures of cognitive capability, and performance in activities of daily living. The actual functioning of all persons lies below the maximum that is possible. How far it lies below is hard to say, but some of the evidence from recovery after stroke or other forms of brain damage suggests that the distance may be considerable; in other words, the normal brain has very large reserves.

Using these three categories, the course of a dementing illness may be represented as shown below.

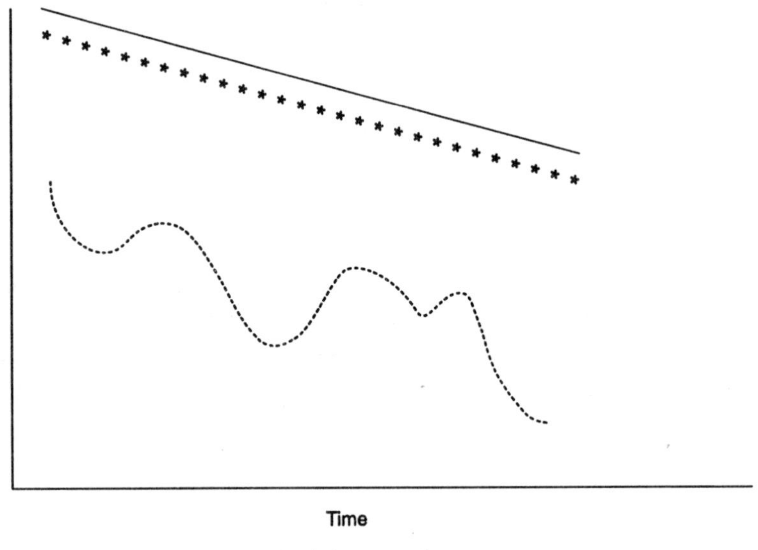

Figure 8.1 Brain structure, brain function and the dementing process

If these ideas are correct in principle (and there is no evidence to suggest that they are not), there are two important consequences. The first is that anyone who assumes that the line representing the third category is tracing the 'true course' of dementia, as directly determined by brain pathology, is making a grave error. In fact this error is made repeatedly, and the findings of medical science are called in as testimony to its truth. The second consequence is that a space is opened up for exploring ways in which a dementing person's actual functioning may be enhanced or diminished through non-neurological factors. These factors may be termed psychological and social-psychological, and of course have their counterparts in functional states in the brain. The theoretical space referred to here is represented on the diagram by the gap between lines 2 and 3.

The person who is missing

Throughout the many debates on the causes and treatment of senile dementia, and indeed in much of the literature on dementia care, certain questions are very rarely asked. Who is the dementia sufferer? What is the experience of dementing really like? How can those who have a dementing illness be enabled to remain persons in the full sense? That they are experiencing subjects, with cognitions, intentions, desires, emotions, there can be no doubt. In the dominant discourse, however, and in some of the subordinate discourses also, dementia sufferers are present largely as an absence. Those who are recognizable as persons are the carers. The dementia sufferers themselves are not; rather, they are defined out of the world of persons, even to the extent of it being claimed, almost literally, that those in the later stages are already dead.

The crudity that results from framing dementia solely in terms set by the dominant discourse is manifest in many of the writings published by the Alzheimer societies, and in many of the standard care manuals. The following is a real example, although no reference is given out of respect for the author's sincerity and commitment to caring. She describes her mother as having been aggressive for a period of 6 months during 'the disease', and attributes this to an affectation of the parts of the brain that supposedly 'control aggression'. She states that she knew her mother was not trying to hurt her; it simply was because her brain was disturbed. But the author goes on to say that the aggression was shown when she and her mother were alone, and never in the company of others. The inconsistencies here are glaring. Bound as she is by the dominant discourse, the author has no possibility of framing her mother as a social and historical being, living in an interpersonal milieu; who deals with her emotional distress in the context of impaired cognitions and impoverished personal resources; and who needs care which takes these things into account.

The exclusion of the person, of which this is typical, is not the whole story. In and amongst the practicalities of care work a different kind of discourse is often generated, in which the personhood of the dementia sufferer is indeed acknowledged. Such a discourse is not underpined by theory, although it moves in a direction that is compatible with an interpersonal psychology of action. Careworkers often seem to operate with a kind of 'doublethink'. On the one hand, there is what they 'know' as standard theory, based on the dominant discourse; and on the other there is what they 'know' through experience. The inconsistency is not unduly troublesome, because it is the latter which informs their actions from day to day, while the official theory is largely bracketed.

The move towards a personal discourse comes about also in another way. Although behaviourism and Reality Orientation have had so great a place, various other kinds of dementia care intervention, more respectful of the dementia sufferer's subjectivity, have also been making their appearance at the margins. Validation Therapy, for example, rests on psychodynamic premises; it suggests that some of those who are in the 'old-old' age range have unresolved developmental and personal issues. As with Erikson's theory of life stages, then, one of two alternatives is possible: the person either deals with the issues (and here the 'therapy' may help), or goes into a dementing process that ends in vegetation (Feil 1982). There are many difficulties here, especially the lack of social considerations, but at least dementia is set into a personal and biographical context. Another form of intervention, so-called Resolution Therapy, has a Rogerian base. It suggests that there is meaning to be found in a dementing person's utterance, however bizarre or confused it may seem to be. The task, then, is to acknowledge the underlying feelings as real, and try to meet the need that is being expressed (Stokes and Goudie 1990). Examples such as these – and there are several others (Jones and Miesen 1991) – point to the beginnings of a reaction to the dominant discourse, an attempt to reinstate the dementia sufferer as a person.

Why, then, is the dementing person so excluded from discourse, and why is there an actual resistance to his or her reinstatement?

One factor, almost certainly, is the prevailing pattern of organizational power and prestige, a pattern that has become deeply entrenched over several centuries. The dominant discourse gives certain professional groups, and psychiatrists in particular, a control of the field. The subordinate discourses provide a place for those with less prestigious roles; both discourse and role are cemented into place. The interests vested in this tacit agreement are numerous: occupational definitions, careers, promotions, investments, publications, the allocation of funding for research. The opening up of a new kind of discourse, one which actually challenges that which is dominant at present, would allocate to psychiatry a far less central role, and elevate the work of humbler professions, particularly the front-line careworkers themselves. The whole structure would be shaken to its core.

The resistance seems to occur also at a psychological level, involving forms of defence which operate below the level of consciousness. The concept of psychological defence, referring to ways in which an individual wards off anxiety, is well known and validated. Perhaps, however, there is another and more powerful tactic: that of collusive defence (de Board 1978; Menzies Lyth 1988). The suggestion here is that in organizations people unwittingly agree together to define their field of work in such a way as to exclude from consideration aspects of that work which would be too painful or anxiety-provoking to take into account. In other words, they create a discourse which systematically defends its participants from psychological threat; and practices develop which are in harmony with the discourse. In the case of dementia the threats principally concern dependency, frailty, loneliness, abandonment, madness, dying and death. In this general area lie some of the darkest fears that confront the human race. It is not surprising that an apparently coherent cluster of discourses has developed around dementia, in such a way as not to engage with these things at all. One token of this whole avoidance is the typical lecture on dementia given to lay persons by an 'expert'. The 'disease', its epidemiology and stages are described; then at some point slides are shown, showing the microstructure of damaged grey matter, and the cross-section of a severely atrophied brain.

THE DEMENTING PERSON REINSTATED

It is clear, then, that both sound theory and good practice require a serious and sustained attempt to understand dementia from within, and hence to create a new discourse, an interpersonal psychology. The fact that no one has yet returned from a demented state to tell us what it is like is certainly a drawback; one which does not apply, for example, to severe depression. Yet this particular 'world of illness' is not wholly inaccessible. Some of its aspects have been described by those in the early stages of a dementing process, urgently demanding that their experience be taken with full seriousness (e.g. Davis 1990). The further recesses, too, can be explored to some extent, when the methods of the poet, the anthropologist and the depth psychologist are combined (see Kitwood and Bredin 1992 for an account based on detailed observational research). Three aspects of a dementia sufferer's experience may be central to the creation of this interpersonal psychology.

1. A loss that can never be 'made good'

Life may be regarded as a process of loss and change, with corresponding 'grief work' to be done. This applies of course to bereavement, but also to losses of many other kinds. In later years loss has a special poignancy, because often there is no prospect of an external restoration. Great personal resources are necessary if this is to be faced without despair (Nemiroth and Colarusso 1985). Those who are dementing may be encountering all these 'ordinary' losses. But in addition they are having to deal with a double loss that is far more devastating: this is their drastic decline in mental capability, and with that a failure in the actual capacity to assimilate the loss. 'Grief work' means making a great readjustment, a reorganization of both life in the world and of inner mental processes, so as to take the new situation into account (Worden 1983). Dementia sufferers can no longer carry out that work. This is why validation therapy, with its emphasis on internal assimilative change, is so often impracticable. The main hope for those who are dementing, in dealing with their losses, is that there will be a coherent external world; with support, comfort, reassurance, stability that can be apprehended directly. For those who have no impairments, memories of good experience and of sustaining relationships can remain, while internal change takes its course. Those who are dementing are more at the mercy of impulse and disorganized fragments of memory. They need a living, palpable interpersonal reality.

2. Actions which fall short of the mark

In the terms set by the dominant discourse, those who have a dementing illness tend to present a range of problems of behaviour. The problems are of course, construed as such from the carers and the professional's point of view. But if we take the dementia sufferer's standpoint, we may usually see these behaviours as actions which are either not recognized, or incomplete because the 'action plan' cannot be retained. Wandering, masturbatory acts, screaming and shouting may, for example, be desperate ways in which a person who is drastically deprived of human contact provides self-evidence that he or she is still alive. Hiding and losing objects may be part of a person's attempt to 'make things safe' when there is an overpowering sense that things are continually being taken away. Some incontinent behaviour may be construed as an enactment of the letting go of hope and self-respect. Aggression may at times be a last bid for recognition by someone who craves desperately for it, but who cannot use acceptable means to gain it. The practical task, then, is to enable a dementia sufferer to retain, as far as possible, his or her sense of agency, and to 'fill out' those pieces of an action which are missing due to cognitive impairment. When a person has very serious deficits in memory and other powers, it may well be that he or she can produce little more than a gesture. The carer's task here is a highly creative one: to acknowledge the gesture, to honour its possibilities, and to enable it to be converted into an action that has meaning in the interpersonal world.

3. On the threshold of unbeing

For many dementia sufferers, especially those who are in the more traditional types of formal care, many hours pass by, day after day, with only the very minimum of human contact. Whatever contact there is may be largely instrumental, concerned with such practical tasks as feeding, clothing and toiletting. In all of this there is very little to replenish the sense of personhood. Someone whose memory is intact can draw on internal processes to retain the sense of personhood in times when contact is scarce or lacking; the continuing thread of selfhood survives in periods of deficit. A dementia sufferer does not have this resource, and so sometimes goes to desperate lengths to stay in the world of persons. If he or she remains passive for too long, the very basis of selfhood is stripped away.

The dementing process has sometimes been likened to a dismantling of the person, a return to a state that resembles, in some respects, that of infancy (Norman 1982). This is valid, but possibly its significance has not been appreciated, because often the dismantling has been construed solely in terms set by the dominant discourse.

We need, rather, to draw on the work of those who have taken a much less mechanical and individualistic approach to understanding our human nature. Winnicott (1965), for example, from a myriad of observations in his clinical work, traced the emergence of personhood in the infant. He suggested that subjectivity arises as fragments of intense experience begin to coalesce, until in due course the continuing thread of selfhood is formed. Also the infant acquires a sense of agency when a gesture meets a facilitating response: one that converts it into an action. In due course these joint actions are taken in, and become the infant's own resource of action schemata. Around these experiences, the infant has to deal with emotional issues that may be near to overwhelming: in particular the many ways in which social living makes the point that he or she is not the centre of the world. The infant, then needs to be held, both literally and psychologically.

In dementia, it seems, processes such as these are invoked again, but in a very different way. As the sense of self sustained by internal processing begins to fragment, it is the environment of others that can alone give continuity. As agency breaks down, it needs to be sustained increasingly by the facilitation which others provide. As emotional traumata continue and intensify, a greater degree of support and holding must be provided by others. Whereas in the case of an infant's development, the carer is doing 'person work' that goes along with a process of neurological maturation, in the case of dementia the carer is working against a process of neurological decline. Whereas, in the case of infants, the intensity of the person-work can become less as time goes on, in the case of dementia the person-work needs to become more intense. Moreover, while nature has prepared instinct-like pathways directed towards the care of infants, it is not at all clear whether this is the case with the care of those who are old and frail; it may be that it is a basically moral concern rather than a biological imperative which motivates the carer's work.

If this is the case, we may understand the course of a dementing illness in a way very different from the standard account, where dementia is seen as the inevitable consequence of an advancing neuropathology. Within a personal discourse, the problem is not simply one of neurological inadequacy. It is, rather, that *the social context failed to provide those conditions that would be necessary for personhood to be retained, and that it failed increasingly as cognitive impairment advanced.* The final state of vegetation, commonly taken to be inevitable, may be reconstrued as one in which an individual has finally lost all hope of, and all means of, reaching out to others and being sustained by them. The self is irreversibly shattered. Personhood has been obliterated, never to return.

THE NEED FOR A PERSONAL DISCOURSE

In this chapter we have touched on many issues related to the discourses of dementia. The crux of the matter is this. We are dealing here with one of the most bewildering and frightening conditions known to humankind: it is so both for those who are afflicted and for those who are closely involved as carers. In the dominant discourse and those which are subordinate to it the dementia sufferer – as a person – has disappeared from view, and the reasons for this are understandable. It is time for a new discourse about dementia to come to the forefront: one which puts personhood at the centre and which spells out what this means for an interpersonal psychology of caring. This discourse would not be subordinate to that produced by medical science; rather, medical science would occupy a certain space within a framework that puts the person first. Some of the key features of this personal discourse are already discernible, and there have been some promising beginnings in practice; a great deal of work is needed to bring this discourse to its full strength.

The creation of a personal discourse about dementia is, then, a challenge on two main grounds. First, it confronts an array of established material and organizational interests; for if the key problems related to the dementing process are to be faced at an interpersonal level, then it is towards that level that the resources need primarily to be directed. Second, it confronts a corresponding array of collusive psychological defences which prevent massive anxieties from being mobilized. A discourse, then, is not simply a matter of ideas and propositions. It is also a matter of organizational power, and of how human beings band together to deal with realities that are often too painful to bear. The dismantling of such a structure, and the replacement of it by something more enlightening and liberating, is a formidable task.

REFERENCES

Albert, M.S. (1982) 'Geriatric Neuropsychology', *Journal of Consulting and Clinical Psychology* 49: 835–50.

Amster L.E. and Kraus, H.H. (1974) 'The relation between life crises and mental deterioration in old age', *International Journal of Aging and Human Development* 5: 51–5.

Bell, J. and McGregor, I. (1991) 'Living for the moment', *Nursing Times*, 87, 18: 45–7.

Blessed, G., Tomlinson, B.E. and Roth, M. (1968) 'The association between quantitative measures of dementia and of senile change in the cerebral grey matter of elderly subjects', *British Journal of Psychiatry* 114: 797–811.

Bredin, K. (1991) 'A Survey of Dementia Care Interventions', Bradford Dementia Research Group.

Davis, R. (1990) *My Journey into Alzheimer's Disease*, Wheaton, Illinois: Tyndale Hall Publishers.

De Board, G. (1978) *The Psychoanalysis of Organizations*, London: Tavistock Publications.

Feil, N. (1982) *Validation Therapy: the Feil Method*, Cleveland, Ohio: Edward Feil Productions.

Folsom, J.C. (1967) 'Reality orientation for the elderly patient', *Journal of Geriatric Psychiatry* 1: 291–307.

Gubrium, J. (1986) *Old-timers and Alzheimer's: the Descriptive Organization of Senility*, London: JAI Press.

Homer, A.C., Honavar, M., Lantos, P.L., Hastie, I.R., Kollett, J.M. and Millard, P.H. (1988) 'Diagnosing dementia: do we get it right?', *British Medical Journal* 297: 894–6.

Hope, J.A. (1986) 'When a new home "cured" the patient's dementia', *Geriatric Medicine* 19: 8–12.

Ineichen, B. (1987) 'Measuring the rising tide. How many dementia cases will there be by 2001?', *British Journal of Psychiatry* 150: 195–200.

Jones, G. and Miesen, B. (1991) *Caregiving in Dementia: Research and Application*, London: Routledge.

Kitwood, T. (1989) 'Brain, mind and dementia; with particular reference to Alzheimer's disease', *Ageing and Society* 9: 1–15.

Kitwood, T. (1990a) 'The dialectics of dementia: with particular reference to Alzheimer's disease', *Ageing and Society* 10: 177–96.

Kitwood, T. (1990b) 'Understanding senile dementia: a psychobiographical approach', *Free Associations* 19: 60–76.

Kitwood, T. and Bredin, K. (1992) *Person to Person: A guide to the care of those with failing mental powers*, Loughton: Gale Centre Publications.

McKhann, G., Drachman, D., Folstein, M., Katzman, R., Price, D. and Stadlan, E.M. (1984) 'Clinical diagnosis of Alzheimer's Disease: report of the NINCDS – ADRDA Working Group under the auspices of the Department of Health and Human Services Task Force on Alzheimer's Disease', *Neurology* 34: 939–44.

Menzies Lyth, I. (1988) *Containing Anxiety in Organizations*, London: Free Association Books.

Nemiroth, N.A. and Colarusso, C.A. (1985) *The Race Against Time*, New York: Plenum Press.

Norman, A. (1982) *Mental Illness in Old Age*, London: Centre for Policy on Ageing.

O'Connor, D.W., Pollitt, P.A., Brook, C.P.B. and Reiss, B.B. (1989) 'The validity of informant histories in a community study of dementia', *International Journal of Geriatric Psychiatry* 4: 203–8.

Roach, M. (1985) *Another Name for Madness*, Boston: Houghton Mifflin.

Rovner, B., Lucas-Blanstein, J., Folstein, M.F. and Smith, S.W. (1990) 'Stability over one year in patients admitted to a nursing home dementia unit', *International Journal of Geriatric Psychiatry* 5: 77–82.

Stokes, G. and Goudie, F. (1990) 'Counselling confused elderly people' in Stokes, G. and Goudie, F. (eds) *Working With Dementia*, Bicester: Winslow Press.

Winnicott, D. (1965) *The Maturational Process and the Facilitating Environment*, London: Hogarth Press.

Worden, J.W. (1983) *Grief Counselling and Grief Therapy*, London: Tavistock Publications.

9 The world of illness of the closed head injured

Paul Bellaby

The sequelae of severe closed head injury share enough of the features of other chronic illnesses to merit the comparison that is the foundation of this book. They also stand out in various ways, partly because of the brain damage involved, partly because of individual, cultural and social factors that typically help form the victim's world of illness.

Sociologists have given little attention to this condition so far. As a result, the chapter has been compiled by rethinking the published findings of clinicians and clinical psychologists (see Richardson 1990 for a recent review). Because the social context of closed head injury is under-researched, original work is presented on a significant category of accidents that often lead to head injury, those of young male motorcyclists. This necessary background material is derived from a survey. It provides a statistical backdrop for the personal experience that stands in the foreground of the chapter.

SOME CLINICAL FEATURES OF CLOSED HEAD INJURY

Closed head injury (henceforth CHI) is brain damage without externally visible lesions. It is commonly the outcome of the rapid acceleration/deceleration of the soft tissue of the brain within the hard shell of the cranium, as may occur in a car, cycle or motorcycle accident or a fall from a horse or down stairs. Commonly, this causes twisting of brain tissue and has effects on the brain in the area at the opposite end of the cranium to where any impact may have occurred. In this way it differs from missile head injury which has specifically focused effects at the point of impact, seldom causing the diffuse damage characteristic of CHI.

The damage may lead to death or to varying degrees of impairment, some transitory. Impairments due to CHI may be physical, including paralysis, spasticity, loss of co-ordination. They may be cognitive, affecting speech, learning and memory. They may also be to do with the emotions or personality: loss of inhibition manifesting as aggression, lability. Typically there is an immediate disturbance of consciousness, which varies from a slight reduction in alertness to deep coma. Among survivors, memory is usually impaired for a period after recovery of consciousness. Needless to say, CHI is often only one of several injuries the accident victim suffers.

The severity of a laceration or fracture can be assessed directly from the evidence to hand. That of CHI must be inferred from the correlation between long-term outcomes and measurements of impairment taken during the acute phase from large samples of the injured. For instance, future disability has been predicted from the length of the post-traumatic amnesia, though more accurately from a battery of indicators of central nervous system damage (Jennett *et al.* 1979). Emotional disturbance is not readily predicted from damage at the point of injury. This suggests that adjustment to CHI is conditioned by such factors as personality or prior social formation and the behaviour of those who care for the injured or are otherwise significant to them (Rutter *et al.* 1984: 105–6). There have been examples of near-complete recovery after severe brain injury, such as those of Colthurst (1990), Keirs (1986) and 'Kim' (MccGwire 1986). These cases imply, as so often in medicine, that the acute phase is not a fully reliable guide for individual prognosis (Roberts 1979: 177). As is the case with disability in other contexts, the social and physical environment in which the victim lives after the acute phase, not the impairment alone, accounts for a considerable part of any disability.

Closed head injury is by no means uncommon. In Britain, there are nine deaths per 100,000 population by this cause, 1 per cent of all deaths (Jennett and Teasdale 1981: 5). Estimates based on acute hospital admissions suggest that the average District Health Authority in England and Wales (of 250,000 population) will encounter the following non-fatal head injuries per annum; some 750 minor, 45 moderately severe and 20 severe (Evans 1987).

THE KINDS OF PEOPLE WHO BECOME CHI VICTIMS

As Rutter *et al.* (1984) point out, it is difficult to establish how much of the condition of a CHI victim is attributable to the sequelae of the injury and how much to the kinds of person who become injured, for pre-traumatic data is usually lacking or unreliable. To a degree the epidemiology of CHI prefigures the worlds of illness that its victims are likely to inhabit.

A study in Olmsted County, Minnesota, based on an extensive medical records system, showed that 274 males and 116 females per 100,000 population suffered head injuries with 'presumed brain involvement' per annum between 1935 and 1974. There was a steep rise for males (to almost 700 per 100,000) in the 16–24 age group (Annegers *et al.* 1980: 913). Jennett and

Teasdale (1981: 5–10) further specify road accidents, especially on motorcycles, as the source of 60 per cent of fatalities from head injury and a high proportion of non-fatal effects.

A survey of 691 young persons' health and life styles in a large part of Norfolk in 1990 (Bellaby and Blaxter 1992; Bellaby and Lawrenson, 1991) allows us to identify the background and characteristics of people who are likely to have accidents of the kind that lead to brain injury.

1. Gender, vehicle use, accidents and risk behaviour

Among males in the achieved sample, 36.2 per cent reported *ever* having had an accidental injury serious enough to require hospital treatment or leave permanent effects. The comparable figure for females was 16.6 per cent. The difference was greater still for accidental injuries that occurred from age 16 onwards. Males reported 260 of these for every 1,000 persons; females 70 for every 1,000 persons. When they were asked where the accident had occurred, males reported more frequently than females in every context but the home: they had had three times as many accidental injuries at school, four times as many in sport, five times as many at work, and seven times as many on motorcycles.

2. Separating the hazards of motorcycles and the risk behaviour of riders

National statistics show that accidents causing death and injury serious enough to require hospital treatment are especially frequent among motorcyclists. For instance, in Britain in 1988 there was a much higher rate of road casualties per 100 million vehicle km on two-wheeled motor vehicles than in cars: more than nine times as many on motorways, and more than 14 times as many on the less safe A-roads (Department of Transport 1989). There are three possible explanations for this:

1 Motorcycles are unstable and more likely to be involved in accidents than other vehicles used on the roads;
2 Motorcycle riders are more vulnerable to serious injury, if they should have an accident, because they are not enclosed as are car or van drivers;
3 Motorcyclists are more 'prone' to accidents, by personality, culture or social circumstances, than other road users.

The first two explanations gain indirect support from official statistics. Only a quarter of motorcycle accidents with casualties involved no other vehicle in Britain in 1989, whereas 35 per cent of car accidents were of this type. Moreover, by far the most common other vehicle to be implicated in motor cycle accidents was the car. No fewer than 63 per cent of all motorcycle accidents with casualties involved a car as well as a motorcycle (Department of Transport 1990). Cars on the road are thus a significant part of the hazard of riding a motorcycle.

Table 9.1 summarizes an analysis of accident rates among those driving cars and riding motorcycles in the Norfolk young persons sample.

Table 9.1 Norfolk survey of young persons
a. Minor accidents with motorcycles and cars
b. Serious accidents with motorcycles and cars and in other contexts

a. Minor accidents with motorcycles and cars
Current regular users who have had a minor accident within the last month before interview

	(1) %	*Base = 100%*
When riding motorcycle	19.6	46
When driving car	4.5	424

b. Serious accidents with motorcycles and cars and in other contexts
Persons driving a vehicle within the last 12 months before interview who *ever* had a serious accident

	(2) *When riding motorcycle* %	(3) *When driving car* %	(4) *In other context Accidents per 1,000 persons*	*Base*
Driving motorcycle only	11.8	N/A	441	34
Driving motorcycle and driving car	12.1	5.5	495	91
Driving car only	N/A	1.5	242	396

The first issue must be whether motorcycles are more likely to be involved in accidents than cars. Official statistics do not allow us to disentangle the probability of having an accident from the probability of being injured or killed in an accident, because they omit accidents that involve no injury (minor accidents). Column (1) (Table 9.1a) represents the percentage of those currently using a motorcycle and/or a car at least once a week who reported a minor accident that occurred on a motorcycle or in a car which they were driving in the month preceding the interview. The rate for motorcycles was almost four times that for cars.

The second issue is how far, given an accident, motorcycles lay their riders open to serious injury more often than cars do their drivers (passengers were omitted from this analysis). Column (2) (Table 9.1b) represents the percentage of those who had ridden a motorcycle in the 12 months preceding interview who had ever had a serious injury as a result of a motorcycle accident; while column (3) gives the corresponding information for car drivers and car accidents. The crucial comparison to be made is between accidents on motorcycles involving motorcycle users in general (whether or not they also used cars) and accidents in cars among those who used only cars. The percentage of the former who had serious accidents was 12.0, and of the latter 1.5. Thus motorcycles proved to be eight times more likely than cars to be involved in serious injury accidents. This disparity is in turn almost twice as great as that involving minor accidents. In other words, motorcycles are more likely to be involved in accidents and more likely to cause their riders serious injury in the event of an accident.

The third issue that the survey allows us to address is the extent to which motorcyclists are a kind of people who are more prone to serious injury than those who drive cars. As Table 9.1b shows, in the 12 months before the interview 91 used both cars and motorcycles. The percentage of these multiple users who had serious accidents in cars was 5.5, three times that of those using cars only. This is consistent with the findings in column (4). Here we tabulate the number of serious accidents per 1,000 persons reported in their life-times by respondents, which did not involve their driving either cars or motorcycles. The rate for those using motorcycles and cars was twice that of those using only cars, and similar to that of those using only motorcycles. In short, the survey data point to the conclusion that those who elect motorcycles as their means of transport are more prone to serious accidents of all kinds than are those who elect cars.

As ever, there are numerous possible confounding factors. Gender is one such. Young women are much less likely to choose motorcycles than men. Males are considerably more prone to accidents in youth and childhood than females. Table 9.2 estimates the rates of car and motorcycle accidents for men and women respectively, and also the extent to which each was prone to serious accidents that did not involve cars or motorcycles.

The table shows differences both between motorcyclists and car-drivers and between men and women. The crucial findings, however, are that both men and women are more likely to have serious accidents on motorcycles than in cars, and that both men and women motorcyclists have a higher accident rate in contexts besides cars and motorcycles than do car drivers. Having established that the preponderance of males among young motorcyclists does not confound the results to date, it is now admissible to point

Table 9.2 Serious injury rates involving car, motorcycle and other accidents, comparing young men and women

	Rate of serious accidents per 100 persons					
	Riding m-cycle	*Other context*	*Base*	*Driving car*	*Other context*	*Base*
Young men	143	417	175	19	314	108
Young women	77	423	52	16	91	186

out that the fact that so many males elect motorcycles may well be an index of their more often being risk-takers than females.

Corroboration of this suggestion comes from responses to questions about drink-driving. Among 266 male drivers and riders, 27.2 per cent said that they had drunk alcohol and driven in the last seven days, and 37.2 per cent that they had ever driven over the blood/alcohol limit. The corresponding figures for women were 12.4 per cent for drink-driving over the last seven days and 15.8 per cent for ever driving when over the limit. As many as two-thirds of the men who had a serious accident on a motorcycle said they had ridden after drink in the last seven days, and more than half of them said they had ever ridden when over the limit.

If gender is one possible confounding factor, age is another. People can and do start riding motorcycles at sixteen, and can only graduate to cars at seventeen. Assuming that age usually involves increasing exposure to driving or riding, it can have two implications with opposite effects for safety. The first is the inexperience which puts the young at risk, and the second exposure to hazards which increases with age. That age is a major factor in serious accidents on motorcycles is abundantly clear from insurance premiums: for instance, in March 1991, a qualified 17-year-old insuring a 500cc Kawasaki comprehensively in East Anglia (a low premium area) would have paid £1,200 per annum, but a 40-year-old doing so would have paid £160 (Norwich Union Insurance Group, personal communication). Inexperience clearly outweighs the effect of increasing exposure. However, there was little difference in the ages of car and motorcycle users in our sample: the average age of regular (once a week plus) riders was 19.9 and of drivers 20.8. Those relatively few who used only motorcycles were younger (18.7), but the difference of one year in the overall averages for cars and motorcycles is almost cancelled out by the fact that motorcyclists could have started a year earlier than car-drivers. As is the case nationally, accidents on motorcycles were most numerous at the age at which most riders were beginning (13 of the 33 for which an age was recorded happened at 17). But car accidents were similarly concentrated by age (that is, experience).

Social class is another possible confounding factor. Since a substantial majority of the sample lived with parents, more than one in six were still in full-time education, and few in employment were sufficiently advanced in their careers to be properly classified by their own occupation, father's occupation was the basis for determining OPCS social class. Among those who were thus classifiable, there was a clear tendency for motorcyclists to have manual fathers. Of young men, 64.5 per cent (N=93) who rode motorcycles in the preceding 12 months, either exclusively or also driving cars, were of social classes IIIM, IV or V. This compares with exactly 50 per cent of the young men who only drove cars (N=188). Young women motorcyclists also had a class bias, though less pronounced: 52.2 per cent of female motorcyclists (N=23) had manual fathers, and only 45 per cent of women who only drove cars.

However, class does not appear to have confounded the comparison between car and motorcycle accident rates. Among males with non-manual fathers who rode motorcycles, 52 per cent had ever had a serious accident, in all circumstances, as compared with 45 per cent of male motorcyclists with manual fathers. Among their counterparts who drove only cars the corresponding percentages were 26 per cent (non-manual) and 36 per cent (manual). Incidentally, though outnumbered almost two to one by men with manual fathers, non-manual men on motorcycles had the same number of serious motorcycle accidents between them as did manual men on motorcycles (8).

Clearly class, like gender and age, serves to select young persons for motorcycling. Having done so, none of these three extraneous variables accounts for the greater tendency of motorcyclists to have serious accidents than car drivers.

The tendency of young men (especially those with manual fathers) to have serious accidents on motorcycles is not wholly attributable to the hazard of using such machines on public roads. To choose a motorcycle at 16 instead of waiting to be eligible for a car licence at 17 and to continue with a motorcycle after 17 are indices of risk-taking behaviour. This behaviour may be partly a matter of personality. It is clearly also an outcome of socio-cultural formation. For some of them, alas, severe closed head injury may ensue.

A CHRONIC ILLNESS IN THE FLUSH OF YOUTH

Any chronic illness becomes interwoven with the life course of the sufferer and also that of family carers. CHI often interrupts biography in youth and preponderantly for males who have been risk-takers.

Prior to assuming adulthood, the adolescent is in an ambiguous position, neither wholly dependent nor wholly independent. However, he or she is the less dependent if male. The male is expected to take risks on his own account or among peers, rather than avoid them as he must when an adult with responsibility for others. Risk-taking by youth may be institutionalized, as in military service. In that case the terms of the licence to take risks are circumscribed. Or risk-taking may be the expected thing – for instance 'skiving' from work – though disapproved of if taken to what elders consider to be excess (Bellaby 1990b). Severe CHI is often the outcome of risk-taking by the young, especially males, as is the high rate of accidental death in civilian life and death in combat. So it is that the situation of the young male helps account for the incidence of CHI.

It also helps account for the aftermath of the injury. For as long as the residual impairments persist, the injured typically become the responsibility of family carers, more often than not mothers or partners (Brooks 1984). When, as is frequently the case, recovery is partial, severe CHI interrupts the life course indefinitely at the point of transition to adulthood; prior to or early in an employment career; before marriage or in a recent marriage; at the threshold of setting up an independent household. The sufferer is thrown back into a degree of dependence on adults that he or she left behind in childhood.

Carers typically find health and social service support to be lacking. In CHI the typical sufferer is anything but typical of the range of patients that the health services are organized to handle. Young males are infrequent users of family practitioner services. Community health services tend to focus on mother and child and the elderly. Such residential care as remains today is overwhelmingly geriatric. Day centres and small bedded units for the rehabilitation of CHI are something of a rarity.

Those closely associated with the victim experience stress after the injury, most acutely in the first few months (Oddy *et al.* 1978). The nature of the illness may lead them to deny its reality. This is largely because the condition is anomalous (cf. Douglas 1966). Victims tend to become moody and aggressive: they are not the same person as their friends and relations knew before the injury. The changes that have come over them are not easy to explain by conventional wisdom. CHI is not degenerative, as are some chronic illnesses in the young (e.g. Huntington's chorea, multiple sclerosis, leukaemia or tuberculosis), but of abrupt onset. The dementia it causes is not inherited. There is simply no ready-made category into which CHI will fit.

TRAJECTORIES OF ILLNESS

If, in observing the progress of CHI, we were to graph changes in physical, cognitive and even emotional functioning, they would describe a curve that falls vertically at the onset of the trauma, and then recovers, with quite a steep slope in the first weeks or months, and later a much lesser gradient, until it becomes asymptotic to the normal trajectory.

Consider how different this time-path is from that of other illnesses. Acute illnesses involve a sharp curtailment of certain functions, followed by a relatively short recovery, which is completed when functioning returns to normal. Chronic illnesses, CHI and also strokes apart, must be divided into those that *gradually* displace the normal life-time curve of functioning downward, but do not hasten its decline, and those that are gradually deteriorative. Perhaps there is a further trajectory for illnesses which are long-standing but leave normal functioning unimpeded: these involve a string of acute episodes.

The trajectory of CHI and individual, cultural and social features of the situation of those surviving CHI

Severe closed head injury abruptly separates individuals from their prior statuses and places them 'on the danger list'. Frequently they are comatose for hours or days. For days or weeks beyond recovery of consciousness, they do not commit anything to memory, and so have no direct knowledge of the circumstances of the injury or its sequel. Recovery of short-term memory is similarly followed by several weeks or months in which cognitive faculties return, but often incompletely and at a retarding rate beyond the first six months to a year after injury. Victims may appear to those who knew them before injury to undergo a change of character. They tend to lose inhibitions and to become labile, libidinous and aggressive. They are also in a highly dependent condition, though of course to a diminishing degree as they recover.

Clearly these conditions have a neurological infrastructure: in his famous case study Luria (1975) referred to the 'shattered world' of one with brain damage. Nevertheless, they have individual, social and cultural features that cannot be simply reduced to brain damage.

Individual features

The temporary loss of awareness which CHI involves implies that the individual cannot give an account of how he or she has arrived at the present condition. Amnesia means that for a period the subject was not present, not part of the world.

Continuing loss of short term memory while still aware of immediate events makes one feel as if dead, because the essence of selfhood is to have a concept of extending backwards and forwards in time and recognizing familiar objects and persons. It is thus crucial to those who recover short-term memory to complete the narrative that post-traumatic amnesia interrupted. In two of the rare autobiographies by the severely head injured (Keirs 1986; Colthurst 1990), the authors use accounts by others to cover for what they cannot remember. They use family's and friends' accounts like a blind person might use the eyes of another.

Severe head injury frequently gives rise to an existential crisis for its victims. This is a state in which a person feels that their life lacks meaning and is beyond their control. In the case of CHI, symptoms of such a crisis include extremes of apathy and depression on the one hand, and aggressive and impulsive behaviour on the other. The first extreme is approached when the individual plays safe in a situation where he or she cannot recognize what is expected of her (cf. entering a room in which only a foreign language is spoken). The second extreme is approached when, instead of playing safe, the individual tries hard to respond to what is mistakenly perceived to be high expectations (cf. acting under the influence of drugs) (Jackson 1987).

Cultural features

One of the few studies of CHI outcomes that have been done with controls makes it clear from the accounts of wives of victims that the existential crisis of CHI is usually much less marked or even absent where patients have only severe physical disability (paraplegia) (Rosenbaum and Najenson 1976).

What is apparently lacking for the victims of CHI which is present for paraplegics is fully-conscious control of the situation. It is a loss which has often been seen as a gain in other times and places. Epilepsy merits some comparison with CHI. Until early modern times it was believed that epilepsy was a sign of possession and conceivably of grace (in spite of Hippocrates' early attack on the concept of the 'sacred' disease, see Temkin 1971). Studies of cultures contemporary with the modern West show that 'going out of one's mind' does not necessarily represent negation of being, but forms a moment in a dialectic impelling one towards rebirth and re-entry into the mundane world as a privileged messenger from a spiritual order that is rarely accessible to ordinary mortals, at least in normal states of consciousness (Lewis 1971). The significance of fully-conscious control over the situation for Westerners bears a definite relation to the emergence of 'possessive individualism' (MacPherson 1962).

A correspondingly individualized approach to health and healing is enshrined in clinical medicine (Young 1980). Solutions to the patient's problems are sought in adjustments of body and mind which are accomplished for or by that individual. The part that may be played in adjustment by changed social relations of the injured person to family carers, peers and employer and by the newly-formed relations with therapists is less likely to be given prominence.

Social features

However, the situation of the CHI victim is social as well as subjective and cultural. It resembles the 'liminality' observed by anthropologists in status-passages. For a period after their separation from their prior status, victims of CHI are upside down, in an indefinite condition, awaiting passage to a new status, which may be one of recovery or of a certain degree of impairment of function.

The concept of liminality was derived from studies of tribal societies: Van Gennep (1960 – originally 1909) synthesized pre-existing ethnography, while Turner (1969) did first-hand research among the Ndembu of what is now Malawi. Van Gennep assimilates numerous rituals with which changes of individual status or states of collective activity are marked, to a three-stage model: separation (from the initial state), transition (between the initial and an improved state) and incorporation (into the new state). The same three stages are plainly seen in the passage from fitness, through severe CHI to recovery or adjustment to impairment. However, there are crucial differences from the tribal model.

The rites of passage in a tribal context are obligatory. Initiation into manhood and womanhood, for example, is normally required of all who attain that approximate age, regardless of physical maturity, and is neither elective, nor (as in the case of the head-injured) occasioned by accident. Rites of passage carry expressive symbolic content as well as being instrumental. Surgery and the rest are routinized technical interventions in the patient's illness, formally void of expressive content. On the other hand, health workers do seek to effect a status passage for the victims of CHI that is not merely a matter of surviving or even being restored to bodily fitness but also a matter of 'healing' or being removed from sickness and restored to normal social rights and obligations.

In view of the balance of similarities and contrasts between status passage involving CHI and rites of passage in tribal societies, the aftermath of CHI is best characterized as liminal-like, or 'liminoid'. The approximate equivalent to liminality, according to Turner (1982) is found in societies not based principally on kinship and affinity as are tribal societies, but based on class relations of production and distribution as is modern capitalist/industrial society.

THE AFTERMATH OF CHI AND THE PERSPECTIVES OF SPECIALISTS AND FAMILY CARERS

Surviving victims are typically treated and cared for by a succession of specialists and thereafter, sometimes permanently, by partners and/or family. Each of these parties, including the victim, is likely to have a different perspective on the injury and its aftermath. In Figure 9.1 below is depicted the passage of victims into and (in most cases) out of the liminoid state. The figure shows how at different stages various specialists are in control, while victim and family carers are present throughout. They are considered to have typically different time-perspectives on the head injury, consisting of a point of entry (*) in the past and a 'horizon' in the future which is indicated by a broken line.

1. Separation

At the point of 'separation', the victim enters surgery. Of all medical specialisms, surgery is most inclined to view the presenting problem as exclusively biomedical, especially with hot (or emergency) as opposed to cold (or elective) operations, where little if anything is learned of the patient as a person and his or her experience of the condition before intervention. The neurosurgeon who admits the victim and operates is largely restricted in practice to securing his or her survival. Thus the couple, 'injury' (of the victim) and 'cure' (of the presenting condition), sets the horizon.

This is not to say that neurosurgeons take no interest in the rehabilitation of their patients. Indeed, many have been active in attempts to ensure that rehabilitation is organized for patients not only while they remain inpatients but also for long after discharge. However, they do not have direct control beyond the post-operative ward.

2. Transition

Assuming that the victim survives, there follows a period of transition in which he becomes a 'novice' under the tuition of nurses, occupational therapists, physiotherapists and others, much like the initiate in a puberty ritual such as Chisungu (Richards 1982), and attempts are made to restore as many as possible of the functions lost due to injury. Recovery of consciousness and memory may be the first steps; followed at an interval by recovery, in part or wholly, of any loss of use of limbs or senses, of speech, and of cognitive skills. This phase takes place within the hospital as a rule and is known as 'acute rehabilitation', though it does not often lead directly to the incorporation of the person into normal life. In this phase, the

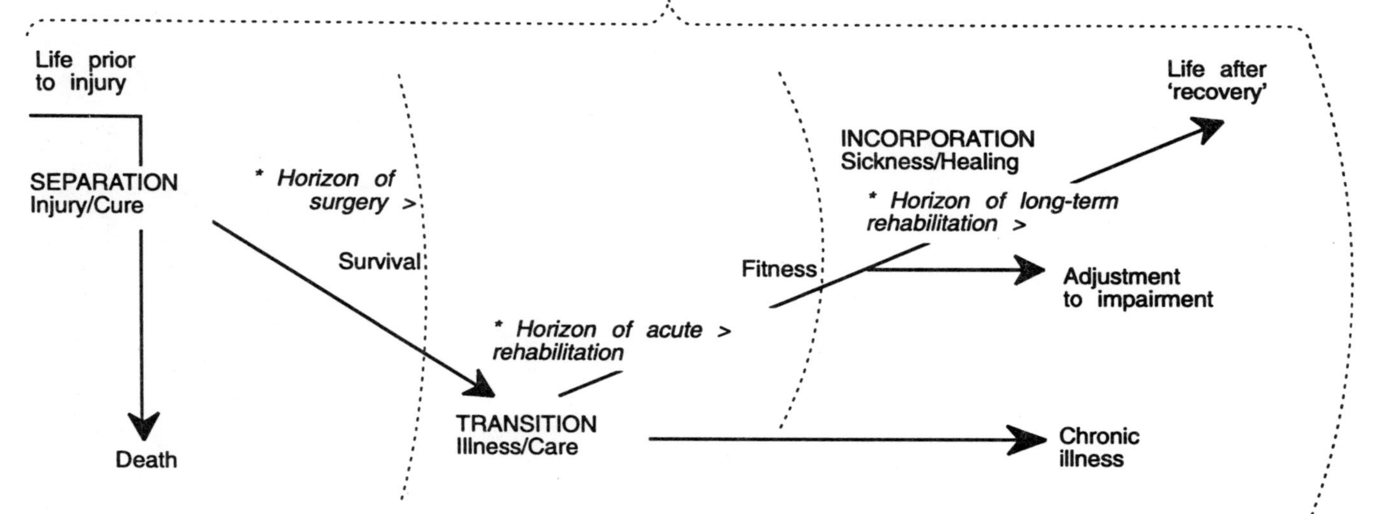

Figure 9.1 The trajectory of closed head injury: the horizons of victim, therapists and carers
Source: Bellaby, P. (1991), reproduced with permission

implications of the injury for the person as a whole – his 'illness' – becomes the focus, and the specialists, with the supervised involvement of family or partner, become 'carers' (as opposed to 'curers'). The horizon of this process is the discharge of the patient from the hospital as 'fit'. In practice, the victims may be discharged to prolonged periods of chronic illness and impairment.

The staff in acute rehabilitation departments are far more likely than the surgeon and his or her team, to learn about the person with the injury – at least through family or partner, and will form a concept of how well that person is likely to adjust to life once incorporated into it, and how much support family or partner are likely to be. They may glimpse, though this is less likely, what kind of person the victim was and what personal relations he or she had before the injury. On the whole, however, the entry point of acute rehabilitation is set to the left (in Figure 9.1) by receiving a survivor from surgery, and its horizon to the right by sending that person out fit or chronically ill.

Specialists here have little control over patients' rehabilitation once discharged to the community. Nor, of course, do they have any control in the surgeon's domain. Cases may thus be handed on from stage to stage with little more co-ordination than case notes allow. The patient's medical record becomes his or her 'life' for practical purposes. This cannot be true for the victim or his or her family or partner, but – while he or she is still an inpatient – non-medical perspectives are likely to be dominated by medical. Nursing staff are best situated to mediate between the long-term perspectives of victim and family carers and the specialized and short-term perspectives of surgeons and other rehabilitation staff.

3. Incorporation

'Incorporation' is the term by which van Gennep understood the restoration of normal life in a status passage. Since tribal societies mark definite changes, usually upward steps in status, by communal ritual, incorporation after closed head injury fits the van Gennep type imperfectly. There is no ritual. The discharge to the community is individual and often routine (marked only by the signing of papers and the departure of an ambulance). Incorporation is not accomplished in a single step, but is a matter of prolonged 'adjustment' to a status that is unlikely to be the same as that prior to injury, far less an improvement. Following Parsons (1979), incorporation normally involves exit from 'sickness' (or the sick role) and the concomitant process of 'healing' usually at the hands of a specialist, which enables the community to accept the patient as a normal citizen. Many victims of severe and moderately severe closed head injury may never leave the sick role or be healed.

It follows that the horizon of long-term rehabilitation is much the most difficult to draw. Victims emerge from acute rehabilitation with a variety of prognoses: from chronic illness through partial recovery to total recovery. There have been attempts to delimit statistically the period of time after injury beyond which further recovery is unlikely or becomes progressively smaller. Such exercises still leave much room for uncertainty in individual cases. Of course, they do not take account of the differences of perspective that surgeons, acute rehabilitators, victims, family carers and psychiatrists might have, and what the effects of such differences among members of the victim's role-set might be on his actual recovery. For outside the hospital context or 'in the community', there is a less clear-cut hierarchical division of labour and much that can be readily supervised in a closed space becomes inaccessible to specialist staff. One perspective, such as that of the neurosurgeon, is much less likely to dominate outside than it did within the hospital. On a day-to-day basis, it is the perspectives of family carers and victim that may carry most weight.

THE INTERPLAY OF TIME PERSPECTIVES AND ITS EFFECT ON THE VICTIM OF CHI

As we have seen, there is sociological value in discovering the various perspectives that members of the CHI victim's role-set have on his or her past, present and future. There may also be therapeutic value. Their time perspectives presumably have a bearing on how they act. In turn they may contribute positively or negatively to the victim's recovery or adjustment to impairment. Figure 9.2 outlines possible relations between recovery and adjustment, and how combinations of active/passive therapy and present/absent social support may influence the victim's progress.

The model implied in Figure 9.2 treats as independent variables, a) recovery of functions lost by brain damage and b) adjustment to a new status. Their separation allows for three possibilities apart from 1. the 'incorporation' through healing depicted in Figure 9.1. These are: 2. adjustment while still impaired (or embrace of the sick role); 3. failure both to adjust and to recover (or a tendency to relapse into social death); and 4. recovery without social adjustment (or becoming a truculent outsider). Figure 9.2 also associates therapy with attempts to promote the recovery of lost functions, and social support with progress towards social adjustment. The therapy the CHI victim receives from the surgeon, and to a large degree that which he gets in acute rehabilitation, is instrumental. Expressive support is left largely to family carers if anyone. We have seen that this support may be problematic. The victim may alienate his or her partner for instance, or return to a state of dependence on a mother.

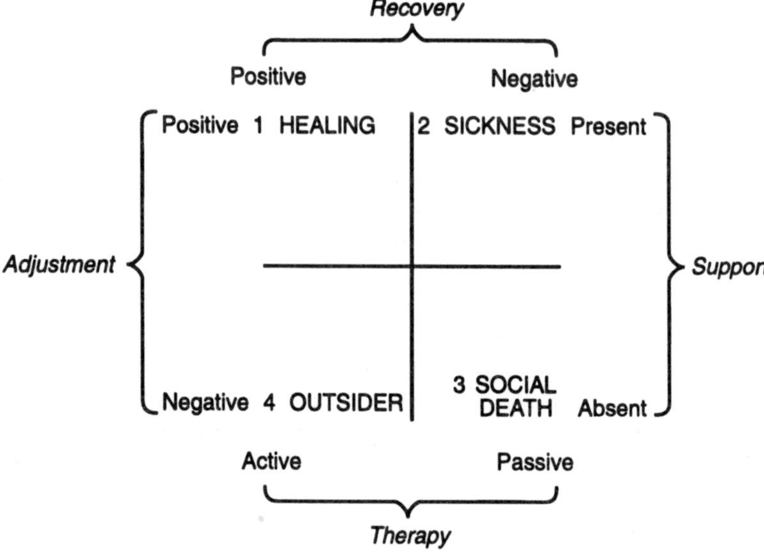

Figure 9.2 Recovery from and social adjustment to CHI
Source: Bellaby, P. (1991), reproduced with permission

Finally, a crucial issue in the outcome of head injury, especially for the young, is return to work. As the biography of 'Kim' (MccGwire 1986) implies, this is a category of patient that may never to return to work, and who, when he or she does return, may find themself in a less demanding job, which is less well paid or has poorer prospects. One ought to ask two questions of this process. The first is why some severe cases return while others do not: do interactions between patient, family carers and therapists have a bearing on this outcome? The second is to what extent the nature of the job itself and the perceptions that employers (and perhaps fellow workers) have of the head injured person can determine the issue. It seems likely, for example, that people employed in a professional or managerial capacity or in a core craft or technical occupation, will find their employer willing to keep their seat warm (as was the case for 'Kim' – a TV journalist of note), while those lacking skills may find that their jobs are not kept open (cf. Bellaby, 1990a). A similar point can be made about how recovery was facilitated by Colthurst's circumstances, since her father, mother and brothers were able to make time so that constant attention could be given throughout her long illness (Colthurst 1990).

CONCLUSION

The aftermath of CHI is frequently chronic illness. However, it differs, subjectively and socially, from most chronic illnesses and disabilities (Blaxter 1976; Anderson and Bury 1988) in a number of ways:

1. It is sudden in onset. In the great majority of cases, there is recovery in the course of time, though in the severer cases, it is almost never complete.
2. CHI, like missile injuries to the brain, falls disproportionately upon young males. Thus, the social incidence of CHI differs from other chronic illnesses. Its impact on the life course is radical, because it commonly strikes close to the first entry to the labour market, to the establishment of an independent household, to marriage and to the first child.
3. CHI not only typically disrupts the victim's expectations in life, it also presents family carers, medical, nursing and paramedical staff and employers with the problem of how to relate the victim's past potential to his or her performance and both to future prospects. There is ample scope for conflict between the assessments each party makes.
4. While other illnesses are commonly seen as either physical or mental, or the product of the mind at work on the body, CHI is hidden in the head, yet is manifested in behaviour that is both physical and mental. In Western culture, individual response to CHI is conditioned by the stress on the autonomy of the self, indicated by fully-conscious and continuous control of the situation, an ability that the closed head injured lack for some or all of their illness.

REFERENCES

Anderson, R., and Bury, M. (eds) (1988) *Living with Chronic Illness*, London: Unwin Hyman.

Annegers, J.F., Grabow, J.D., Kurland, L.T. and Laws, E.R. (1980) 'The incidence, causes and secular trends of head trauma in Olmsted County, Minnesota', *Neurology* 30: 912–19.

Bellaby, P. (1990a) 'What is a genuine sickness? The relation between work discipline and the sick role in a pottery factory', *Sociology of Health and Illness* 12: 47–68.

Bellaby, P. (1990b) 'To risk or not to risk? Uses and limitations of Mary Douglas on risk-acceptability for understanding health and safety at work and road accidents', *Sociological Review* 38: 465–83.

Bellaby, P. (1991) 'Histories of sickness: making use of multiple accounts of the same process', in S. Dex (ed.) 'Life and work history analyses: qualitative and quantitative developments', *Sociological Review Monographs* 37, London: Routledge.

Bellaby, P. and Blaxter, M. (1992) *The Health and Life Styles of Norfolk Youth*, Centre for Health Policy Research Report Series No. 7, University of East Anglia.

Bellaby, P. and Lawrenson, D. (1991) 'Accidents and youth: deconstructing the stereotype of the young tearaway', *British Sociological Association*, Annual Conference, Manchester (available from authors).

Blaxter, M. (1976) *The Meaning of Disability*, London: Heinemann.

Brooks, N. (1984) 'Head injury and the family', in N. Brooks (ed.), *Closed Head Injury: Psychological, Social and Family Consequences*, Oxford: Oxford University Press.

Colthurst, G. (1990) *Fighting Back*, London: Methuen.

Department of Transport (1989) *Road Accidents. Great Britain 1988: the Casualty Report*, London: HMSO.

Department of Transport (1990) *Road Accidents. Great Britain 1989: the Casualty Report*, London: HMSO.

Douglas, M. (1966) *Purity and Danger: an Analysis of the Concepts of Pollution and Taboo*, London: Routledge & Kegan Paul.

Evans, C. (1987) *Headway*, Conference, Sheffield, 5–6 November.

Jackson, M. (1987) *Headway*, Conference, Sheffield, 5–6 November.

Jennett, B., Teasdale, G., Braakman, R., Minderhoud, J., Heiden, J. and Kurze, T. (1979) 'Prognosis of patients with severe head injury', *Neurosurgery* 4: 283–9.

Jennett, B. and Teasdale, G. (1981) *Management of Head Injuries*, Philadelphia: F.A. Davis.

Keirs, J. (1986) *A Change of Rhythm*, Nottingham: Headway.

Lewis, I.M. (1971) *Ecstatic Religion*, Harmondsworth: Penguin.

Luria, A.R. (1975) *The Man with a Shattered World*, Harmondsworth: Penguin.

MccGwire, S. (1986) *Kim's Story: a Fight for Life*, London: Harrap.

MacPherson, C.B. (1962) *The Political Theory of Possessive Individualism*, London: Clarendon.

Oddy, M., Humphrey, M. and Uttley, D. (1978) 'Stresses upon the relatives of head-injured patients', *British Journal of Psychiatry* 133: 507–13.

Parsons, T. (1979) 'Definitions of health and illness in the light of American values and social structure', in E. Jaco and E. Gartley (eds) *Patients, Physicians and Illness*, third edition, London: Collier Macmillan.

Richards, A. (1982) *Chisungu: a girls' initiation ceremony among the Bemba of Zambia*, second edition, with an introduction by J. la Fontaine, London: Routledge.

Richardson, J.T.E. (1990) *Clinical and Neuropsychological Aspects of Closed Head Injury*, London: Taylor and Francis.

Roberts, A.H. (1979) *Severe Accidental Head Injury*, London: Macmillan.

Rosenbaum, M. and Najenson, T. (1976) 'Changes in life patterns and symptoms of low mood as reported by wives of severely brain injured soldiers', *Journal of Consulting Clinical Psychology* 44: 881–8.

Rutter, M., Chadwick, O. and Shaffer, D. (1984) 'Head injury', in Rutter, M. (ed.), *Developmental Neuropsychiatry*, London: Churchill Livingstone.

Temkin, O. (1971) *The Falling Sickness*, second edition, Baltimore: Johns Hopkins University Press.

Turner, V. (1969) *The Ritual Process*, London: Routledge & Kegan Paul.

Turner, V. (1982) *From Ritual to Theatre*, New York City: Performing Arts Journal Publications.

Ván Gennep, A. (1960) *The Rites of Passage*, translated by M.B. Vizedom and G.L. Caffee, London: Routledge & Kegan Paul.

Young, A. (1980) 'The discourse of stress and the reproduction of conventional knowledge', *Social Science and Medicine* 14B.3: 133–46.

10 On knowing the patient: experiences of nurses undertaking care

Martha MacLeod

INTRODUCTION

During shift-to-shift hand-over reports on Scottish surgical wards, it is not uncommon to hear nurses say about a patient, 'He's better in himself'. This phrase, recorded in field notes during a recent study of excellent, experienced, surgical nurses, was found to point towards the ways in which nurses are attuned to the patients' experience of illness, recovery and hospitalization.

In the study, nurses talked about how a patient was feeling 'in himself', to express how the person was feeling overall, despite the presence of clinical problems such as urinary retention, constipation or a wound infection. Frequently, the nurses would ask the patient, 'How are you in yourself?' and at other times would infer from the patient's countenance and actions that he was feeling better overall. It would seem that asking 'How are you in yourself?' takes the common, polite question of 'How are you?' one step farther. This is not a request for a surface answer. The question indicates a genuine interest and an invitation to be open. The nurse wants to know how the patient is really feeling. Nurses also ask patients' families, 'How do you find her in herself?' This too, invites openness, for the family to say what they are noticing about their family member's experience and recovery. It acknowledges that the family can recognize subtle distinctions in the patient's demeanour, and it invites them to share it with the nurse. These commonly used phrases point towards how nurses understand the patient as a person. In so pointing, the illness and trappings of hospitalization are not trivialized. They are, instead, transparent as the nurse looks at the person and sees how they are – in themselves. Patients are also encouraged to know and understand themselves differently from the nurse's question. They are invited to understand that they can be 'better in themselves' while in a stressful and possibly frightening situation following surgery. Their current feelings of illness and the effects of surgery are reframed as being temporary; secondary to themselves. 'He's better in himself' captures many of the ways in which nurses know a patient recovering from surgery.

In the research study, the everyday experience in nursing practice of ten excellent, experienced Scottish ward sisters (head nurses) was explored with a view to understanding how that everyday experience contributes to the development of expertise (MacLeod 1990). It became evident in the study that knowing patients and being attuned to patients' experience of illness and hospitalization were embedded in the ward sisters' moment-by-moment practices of helping individuals towards recovery whilst making the ward work for all the patients.

In this chapter, I will specifically examine the ways in which the ward sisters come to know the 'person' of the patients in their care, how that knowledge develops and is modified, and how knowing the person enables the nurse to help the patient towards recovery. Notably, the focus is on the ways in which nurses, in their everyday, moment-by-moment experience with patients, their families and other health care workers, come to understand the experience of illness and hospitalization. By means of this exploration I will argue for a different understanding of nurses' experience, particularly in relation to patients' experience of illness. I will suggest that the nurses' taken-for-granted practices through which they know their patients reveal the intersubjective and relational nature of experiencing illness and recovery. Further, we will see that different features of the lived experience of illness, recovery and hospitalization show up in the shared background practices and language of patients, their families and nurses.

PATIENTS AND NURSES – IN SEPARATE WORLDS OR TRAVELLING TOGETHER?

Can nurses and patients share the experience of illness? How do nurses know the patients and understand their illness experience? Implicit in these questions are ways of understanding the notions of experience and knowledge.

Nursing and medical literature have long been characterized by a reification of objectively determined, formal, scientific knowledge. As Freidson (1986) suggests, formal knowledge is the hallmark of the professions. The subject of research and teaching, formal knowledge is:

> formalized into theories and other abstractions, on efforts at systematic, reasoned explanation, and on justification of the facts and activities believed to constitute the world.
>
> (Freidson 1986: 3)

Despite the realities of clinical practice in which many areas are imprecisely known or uncharted, formal knowledge is valued by medicine and nursing as the form in which illness and disease is best depicted. Medicine has long considered illness as an objective phenomenon to be diagnosed and treated. Nursing on the other hand, claims to attend to peoples' illness experience (e.g. Benner and Wrubel 1989). Nursing's imperative is to foster 'the physical and psychological well-being of persons, especially when ill, by caring for them in personal relationships' (Bishop and Scudder 1990: 171).

Notwithstanding its commitment to the human experience of illness, nursing also values the generation of formal knowledge over other, less scientifically credible ways of knowing (Carper 1978; Meleis 1985). Studies of patients' experience of illness have reflected an assumption that experience is 'aggregates of distinct, separable perceptions, conceptions and skills' (Van Manen 1977: 216). Nursing studies of such phenomena as pain (Seers 1987; Closs 1991) or wounds (Wilson-Barnett and Batehup 1988) have consistently overlooked or paid scant attention to the meaning for the patient of these experiences. Experience is measured and objectively assessed, frequently through observational measures or subjective responses to objectively set questions.

In an attempt to attend to the meaning of illness for patients, a small but growing number of studies are investigating subjects' personal knowledge. For example, Baker (1989) sought knowledge of patients' experience of post-operative recovery and Brown (1986) studied patients' experience of being cared for by nurses. Notably, these studies and others like them seek to understand the phenomenon from the subject's point of view. I would suggest that an assumption underlying these studies is that experience is within the realm of personal knowledge and as such, it is highly personal, subjective and idiosyncratic (Carper 1978). In the same way that experience is understood to be an inner, subjectively-held phenomenon, so too in these studies, meaning is considered to be subjectively held. Thus, a dichotomy between subjective and objective knowledge exists in these studies of personal experience, as well as in the objective studies of experience.

The dichotomy is also evident in several studies which explore the world of illness and medical care (Strauss *et al.* 1985; Corbin and Strauss 1985; Conrad 1987). These studies move quickly from an analysis of the subjective experience of the actors: patients and caregivers, to an explanation of the underlying social processes.

While all such studies make important contributions to our understanding of illness and health care, they leave some important gaps. Among the gaps is the relative inattention to the situational, temporal and relational nature of knowledge and experience.

Following Heidegger (1962), Polanyi ([1958]1962) Merleau-Ponty (1962) and Dreyfus (1980), Benner (1984, 1989) argues for a different understanding of experience and knowledge, one which does not follow these objective/subjective lines. She proposes a distinction between knowing which is embedded within a particular situation and knowing which is formal and abstract. The distinction is between 'knowing how' and 'knowing that'. For nurses, practical knowledge, knowing how, is knowledge derived from experience, from the day-to-day business of caring for patients. This knowledge is not idiosyncratic, personal knowledge, because it is shared in language and practices. Experience, in this view, is not purely subjective: it is already commonly shared in the world. Meaning is not subjectively held to be negotiated by the self, but is already there in our language and everyday practices.

These differing ways of understanding knowledge and experience imply differing possibilities of how nurses might know patients and understand the experience of illness. Many studies of patients' experiences (e.g. Webb 1986) highlight aspects of those experiences of which nurses appear to be unaware. People writing of their illness experiences also note that nurses and other health professionals frequently do not share or understand their experience (e.g. Saxton and Howe 1988). At the same time, they comment on the extraordinary understanding shown by some individuals.

Studies which are predicated upon a view that experience is held by the individual or as a phenomenon to be objectively examined, give the appearance that patients and health care workers are in separate experiential worlds. However, there are other studies and descriptions of experience (e.g. Sacks 1985; Benner and Wrubel 1989; Kesselring 1990) which show a different view of how patients and health care workers can move together in the experience of an illness. They show how experience and meanings can be shared. This view is echoed by practising nurses who talk about how they 'travel together with patients' through the illness experience (Hosang pers. com. 1991).

Before pursuing the questions of whether patients and nurses exist in separate worlds or travel together, I will briefly describe the research which forms the basis of this chapter.

THE APPROACH TO THE STUDY

The interpretative research upon which this chapter is based was conducted over an eleven-month period with ten 'excellent, experienced' Scottish nurses. The intent was to uncover the nature of experiencing nursing practice.

The interpretative approach informing this research and discussion can be traced to the philosophical work of Heidegger (1962), who suggests that peoples' actions and experience are not a combination of objective properties and subjective beliefs, feelings and perceptions. He proposes instead, that human existence is better understood to be historical and intersubjective in nature. Our language and taken-for-granted actions show that we cannot be disconnected from our surroundings, from each other and from the influence of time. Studies which concentrate on subjective beliefs or objective properties fail to capture this complexity of human experience.

One of Heidegger's examples illustrates the everyday skilful coping in taken-for-granted experience. When we open a door, we are not aware of turning the doorknob, we are only aware of the doorknob when it sticks. When the doorknob sticks we attempt to un-stick it, and it is only when that does not work that we may need to think about the specific properties of the doorknob itself. Heidegger argues that what needs study before the problem of knowing is everyday being-in-the world, as 'much if not most characteristic human activity is not guided by conscious choices, and not accompanied by aware states of mind' (Magee 1987: 260). It would follow then that much of everyday experience is overlooked and taken for granted because it is skilful coping in the midst of an ongoing situation. Unless a problem develops or a doorknob sticks, we remain unaware of the skills and knowledge essential to this coping. The coping is not only with the more physical aspects of our practices, it also involves their human and interactional nature.

Studies which use hermeneutic phenomenology (e.g. Benner 1984; Kesselring 1990) seem to be more successful at capturing the complex nature of experience, illness and nursing practice. For example, Benner's (1984, 1989) research reveals: the ongoing context of practice of which tasks are but a part; the goals and meaning of practice; the knowledge and decision-making skills required to care for patients in an appropriate and timely manner; the interconnected nature of the individual and the social world. Through this interpretative approach the richness and complexity of nursing experience, practice and knowledge can be revealed.

The study

Insights on the nurses' experience in everyday practice were sought through an eleven-month period of field work which consisted of participant observation, a group interview and three reflexive interviews with each nurse.

The nurses,[1] identified by the hospitals' Directors of Nursing Services, met criteria adapted from Benner (1984) to identify expert nurses. They were reputed to be 'excellent, experienced, surgical nurses'. Eight were ward sisters; the other two, staff nurses, fulfilled part of a ward sister role. They had from six to thirty-three years of nursing experience. Locating experience and excellence in clinical practice at this position is not unusual in the

National Health Service. The ward sister is generally thought to be the 'repository of clinical expertise' (Lathlean 1987: 16).

Two principles were touchstones throughout the research. First, my attention was focused on the nurse-in-practice, not on the nurse removed from a context, nor on the context without the nurse. Second, I endeavoured to 'keep close' to experience, to continually ask while in the field and during interpretation, 'What does this mean about experience?'.

A hermeneutic interpretation

Hermeneutics is an 'attempt to make clear, to make sense of an object of study' (Taylor 1971). In this study, the interview transcripts and field notes were treated as text, or text analogues and a hermeneutic interpretation carried out with them (Gadamer 1975, Ricoeur 1979, Rabinow and Sullivan 1979).

In this approach, the meaning of an action or text (or text analogue) does not rest only in the writer, actor or speaker, nor in the interpreter alone, but is constituted in both. The interpretation sought was not the sisters' interpretation of their own situation, nor was it merely mine. Instead, I aimed to bring to light what the sisters already understood about their experience and practices, but in a new way, in a new interpretation, one beyond their own.

KNOWING THE PATIENT

When the interviews and field notes were closely examined, the phenomenon of experience was found to be more complex than it is frequently described in the research literature. Two senses of experience were found: 1. experience as a resource or entity, something which the person had or could gain; and 2. experience as an ongoing process, the process of experiencing. These two senses of experience were found to be in continual interplay, with experience as a resource growing out of, informing and being changed by the process of experiencing. Experience was found to be grounded in concrete activities, situated in time and place. The ongoing process of experiencing was found to be inextricably bound to the ward sisters' moment-by-moment practices. That is, the everyday work of being with and caring for patients was also, for the ward sisters, the process of experiencing the patients and experiencing nursing practice. As they went about their daily work, the ward sisters were attuned to experience: to the experience of patients, to the experience of families, to the experience of other health care workers and to their own experience.

This process of experiencing has been characterized as an inextricably intertwined process of noticing, understanding and acting (MacLeod 1990).

Concomitantly, this process was also found to be the ongoing process through which the ward sisters practise nursing. It is evident in the relational and contextual nature of their practices. The qualitative character of this process seems to contribute to the sisters' practice being complex, multifaceted, goal directed and centred on the patient. Noticing was found to be more than seeing or hearing or assessing: it is a process of interpretation. Understanding is more than a surface knowing or recognition: it is a deep comprehension of meanings inherent in a situation. And acting goes beyond mere behaviour or deployment of skills: it is practising in a concrete situation. Through their concerned, involved stance in a situation, the sisters notice salient features, understand their meaning and act, caring for the patient.

Understanding appears to be comprised of both theoretical knowledge and practical knowing. The field notes and interviews reveal knowing the patient to be an integral part of moment-by-moment practising. The sisters talk about knowing the patient as being a central part of their nursing practice.

> *Sr Hanna*: And I felt that you have to get to know patients and once you get to know them, then you can nurse them better. So to me just getting to know them and knowing what was going to happen to them was part of nursing skill.
>
> (Int. 8–3: 22)

The ward sisters told of learning about the meaning of illness from patients and without exception, said that patients were their greatest teachers. Importantly, all of them said that knowing the patient was necessary in order to care for them.

This contention of practitioners, that knowing the patient is a central part of nursing practice has been explored by Benner *et al.* (1991) in expert nursing practice. It is a recurring theme in the nursing literature. For example, Marram Van Servellen (1982) suggests that knowing the patient is necessary in order to provide individualized nursing care. Among others, May (1991) identifies knowing the patient as a component of nurse-patient relationships.

For the ward sisters, knowing the patient is not a simple, nor unitary phenomenon. It includes becoming familiar with many of the patient's 'everyday habits, practices and preferences as well [as] his or her usual demeanour and self-presentation' (Benner and Wrubel 1989: 392). It also includes learning how people respond to hospitalization, the procedures and the surgery they undergo. The ward sisters speak of the importance of the family in knowing the patient. Frequently, families help the nurses to recognize subtle changes in patients (Benner and Wrubel 1989: 392). Working with the family, the ward sister comes to know how they support and care for their ill member and gains their assistance in helping the patient towards recovery.

As in all of the other practices of the ward sisters, knowing the family is situated in time and place. They know the patients and their families in the context of the patients' admission to the surgical ward, illness, surgery and recovery process. When the ward sisters talked about memorable experiences with patients, the temporal sense of the narrative related to the patients' course of illness and stay on the ward. This temporal sense was also evident in shift-to-shift hand-over reports and other aspects of the ward sisters' practices. As the ward sisters work with patients and their families, they get to know the patients and modify that knowledge within the context of helping the patients towards recovery from surgery.

Getting to know the patient: respecting and trusting the person

From the time of admission, the ward sisters foster the respect and trust of the patient and through their practices, show their respect for and trust of the patient. A kind of 'reciprocal trust' (Thorne and Robinson 1988) is evident in the relationships between the ward sisters and their patients.

Throughout their daily work: co-ordinating care, making rounds, giving medications, dressing wounds, making beds and responding to patients' requests, the ward sisters get to know their patients.

> *Sr Hanna*: It's mostly by personal contact and by chatting to them. [...] Well, the main thing for me is doing their wounds. You know, making their beds .... As [...] you make their beds if they're sitting beside, you chat to them. And you know, casually find out about the families and you know, how they manage at home and this sort of thing.
>
> (Int. 8–3: 23)

Chatting to patients outwardly appears to be simple and innocuous, centring around social talk. However, for the ward sisters, it has a focus.

> Sr Hanna goes to give the Metroniazole suppository to Mrs Prior (the medication route was changed the previous evening as Metroniazole is less nauseating by suppository), Mrs Prior looks bright and says, 'I feel good'. She says she's been thinking about doing her laundry, and that she is concerned about her husband boiling it. As she gives the suppository, Sr Hanna listens and shares a story of when she was in hospital having her youngest baby and her husband boiled the jeans, long before boiled jeans were in style.
>
> (W8D3: 6)

This excerpt speaks of how the ward sisters are present with patients, acknowledging and preserving their sense of being persons, as well as being patients. The ward sisters touch their patients' experiences, by the timing and pacing of their actions, by listening and by sharing themselves and their own experiences. Through this conversation, this 'chat', Sr Hanna comes to know something of Mrs Prior's home supports, and her level of comfort with how her husband is managing. Sr Hanna also comes to know more about Mrs Prior's experience of this medication. The chat helps them through an intimate, potentially embarrassing nursing procedure. By their actions and presence, the ward sisters show patients that it is all right to share the little but possibly important things.

In addition to coming to know patients through conversation, nurses come to know patients by being present with them. The nature and pattern of nursing work, in which nurses are with patients over continuous periods, sets up this possibility. They witness patients' struggles with illness, technology and recovery. Frequently, it is difficult for the ward sisters to put what they know about being present with patients into words. They talk of coming to understand patients and the ways in which individuals experience illness and recovery by 'just being with' patients and 'seeing how they are', by 'caring for' and 'just looking after' patients.

The ward sisters talk about how patients 'tell you', even when they cannot communicate verbally and are on artificial ventilation machines.

> *Sr Dunn*: You can tell an awful lot just by looking at your patient. Or holding their hand, their colour or how warm or cold they are or speaking to them, of their reaction. There's an awful lot you can tell from your patient, from observing the patient without any machines at all.
>
> (Int. 4–3: 36)

The ward sisters tell about how they come to notice and understand the meanings of the small gestures and facial movements of people who are unable to speak. They are attuned to the patients and notice small changes in the normal pattern of sounds, for instance, when someone's breathing pattern is changing. They are familiar with the normal smells of wounds and notice almost imperceptible changes. As the ward sisters develop expertise, the skill of their bodies give them access to a situation with less effort and increased sensitivity (Benner and Tanner 1987).

The ward sisters know the families as offering a 'tremendous amount of support for the patient' and a fund of information 'which you can or cannot tap', depending upon how much you value them (Int. 7–1: 18).

> *Sr Grant*: ... Well, I found out a great deal about the patient himself. What his personality was like, from his wife ... She said things like, '... he's very stubborn', 'And [...] he's easily disheartened'. Which were two things that we hadn't really picked up on because we didn't know him very well. He

> was only supposed to be in for four days here; arrived the afternoon before his operation so we had little opportunity [...] to find out what he was like.
>
> (Int. 7–1: 18)

All of the ward sisters walk around to the patients' beds and talk with the families during visiting hours.

> *Sr Grant*: My opening statement is always, 'How have you been finding him?' Because generally that yields worries and also a good assessment of really how the patient is. Because they know the patient best.
>
> (Int. 7–2: 18)

Asking the family 'How have you been finding him?' not only gives the ward sister insight into the patient, but also indicates a respect of the family's interpretation of the patient's recovery. It opens the way for dialogue about their understanding and concerns. The ward sister can learn more about their experience of illness in their family member. Importantly, when the family tells the ward sister about what they are noticing about the patient and what it means, dialogue ensues. Both families and the ward sisters revise their interpretation or have new confidence in it and gain new insights.

The continuous nature of nursing work places the ward sisters in a position to know patients and their families differently than the way in which doctors and other health care workers know the patients.

> *Sr Dunn*: The doctors are coming round once a day, twice a day standing at the bottom of a patient's bed. They're not *with them*, while the girls that are on a full shift, you know seven hours, and seeing their relatives coming … .
>
> (Int. 4–1: 27)

The continuity afforded by their pattern of work enables the ward sisters to come to understand the patients' experience of hospitalization and recovery. The benefits of this are seen especially when patients return.

> *Sr Grant*: I think there's a positive advantage for the patients to see a familiar face. Cause they KNOW that you know what they went through last time. And I think there's some security in seeing someone that you know.
>
> (Int. 7–2: 14–15)

The way in which nurses know the patients is constrained as well as facilitated by the context of their knowing. The ward sisters say they do not get to know the majority of patients as people because most are on the ward only for a short period of time. However, people who have major surgery, who are admitted repeatedly, or who have problems with recovery, are the patients whom the ward sisters talk of having the privilege of knowing well.

'He's coming along as expected' – knowing the person in the context of recovery

Through their experience of nursing many surgical patients, the ward sisters come to understand a range of 'normal' recovery patterns for most types of surgery. They come to recognize signs of people feeling better and know what kinds of actions help that process. For example, Sr Fraser describes her knowing of patients' experience when intravenous and nasogastric tubes are removed. 'As one or another of the bits and pieces around them are coming down they feel better in themselves' (W6D5: 7).

The ward sisters compare one person's response to how others in their experience have responded.

> *Sr Baxter*: I saw before I went to her that she was looking smarter ... she'd had make up on. [...] There are some people that don't wear make up and you can see it. [...] It's the way they look. They just *look* better.
>
> (Int. 2–2: 19)

The ward sisters have a finely-tuned knowledge of individuals' physiological responses to anaesthesia, surgery and recovery in the light of normal patterns. Sr Ellis reminds the resident doctor of Mr Meek's past experiences of having low blood pressure following anaesthesia. 'It's part of Mr Meek's pattern' (W5D2–2: 8). With her extensive experience caring for patients with peripheral vascular disease, Sr Aitkin has come to understand the many ways patients experience vascular limb pain and pain following amputation. She gets to know patients' patterns of pain and their response to it. When a patient is in an unusual amount of pain following an amputation, Sr Aitkin persists in getting the resident to bivalve the cast to relieve a build-up of pressure, despite no obvious signs it was needed. 'I've known her for a long time. ... She had pain' (W1D5: 11).

Not only do the ward sisters become knowledgeable about the physiological nature of the effects of surgery, they also understand something of the meaning to people of the assaults of surgery. Sr Dunn has a well-developed knowledge of how people experience chest wounds. Her understanding begins with knowing the normal range of pain people have related to the wound and the chest tubes, the materials used for dressings and how they work with different skin types, how different adhesives stick, how skin reacts, what to do if there is a problem and how to avoid it. It does not stop there, however. Through long experience in helping individuals learn to live with chronic purulent chest wounds, Sr Dunn has developed an appreciation of the various meanings the wound has to each of the patients she works with.

The ward sisters come to know a range of patterns and sometimes talk about a 'type' or 'kind' of person. For example, in discussing the plans to send a patient with aesophageal cancer home with his only means of nutrition through tube feedings, Sr Fraser comments, 'He doesn't strike me as the type of man that's going to be able to cope' (Int. 6–3: 4). She has seen how he has coped so far with having the tube, refusing to have anything to do with it. Based on her knowledge of other patients and how they have coped, she anticipates that he will have difficulty. The ward sisters speak of seeing the patients' character through such everyday ways of being such as how they move, what they do for themselves, how they talk about goals for when they go home and how they are supported in a family. The ward sisters get to know who will actively work towards recovery and who will likely have more difficulty.

It could be construed that much of the ward sisters' knowing is imbued with certainty, with regularity rather than difference. However, that is not the case. By constantly comparing an individual's response to illness and recovery to their knowledge of others' responses, the ward sisters not only learn about the individual but also keep their practices and knowing in question.

Much of their understanding of the experience of illness stems from sharing the language and culture of their patients. But what happens when the language or culture is different? In the study, there were very few patients who were not of the same British culture. Sr Grant puzzles over the pattern of complaining and concern of Mr Singh, an Asian patient. She notices that he seemed to be 'preoccupied with his aches and pains generally' (W7D1: 17). In a report to her staff nurse, she recognizes that his response is unusual and there might be something more going on:

> 'I'm not experienced in this: I don't know if it is an ethnic thing or him: I think it might be him. His sons are calling him a hypochondriac and are getting impatient with him.'
>
> (W7D2:4)

Sr Grant keeps her knowledge in question over the next three days as she tries to understand Mr Singh's anxiety, physical complaints and reluctance to go home. She gradually ascertains that there are issues in the dynamics of the family which she cannot address. Although she listens for them, she does not pick up distress or any 'cries for help' from the family. Sr Grant does, however, identify Mr Singh's main complaint as constipation and helps him and his wife to explore ways in which they can cope with this problem themselves at home.

Together in a historical time and place, the ward sisters and patients share a history. By virtue of the moment-by-moment practices by which the ward sisters help patients move through the process of surgery and recovery they get to know each other. With patients, the ward sisters assume a stance towards the possibilities of the future, possibilities which they realize with the patient because of their knowledge and shared history with the patient.

'She's back to her old self' – knowing the 'real' person

On the one hand, the ward sisters continually make comparisons amongst different people's responses to illness and surgery. On the other hand, they continually compare an individual's responses over time.

'She's back to her old self'. A patient who has had a rough post-operative course is beginning to show some of the sense of humour which she showed to the nurses before her operation. With experience, the ward sisters come to understand the profound effects that illness and surgery can have on people. They cannot be adequately captured by a list of attributes and adjectives. Instead, the ward sisters speak of the effect of illness by talking about the person which they know in crisis as not being the 'real one'. 'They're different people' (Int. 4–2: 32). That is, the person they know in the hospital is not the same person as the well one who goes about their daily life outside of this context. Returning to her 'old self' through recovery speaks of an emphasis on the temporary nature of illness and the goal of recovery, for the person to return to normal.

When the ward sisters are faced with a person who is having problems in recovering, they attempt to find and draw on the resources of the 'real' person. Sr Grant, faced with a tearful Mr Singh just hours before he was to go home, suggests that he not go home in pyjamas.

Sr Grant: You have a lot of dignity. Going home in clothes lets you go out with dignity. You're not an old man.

Mr Singh: I feel like an old man.

Sr Grant: You're in the prime of your life and you have a long time to go. Wearing clothes going out of here shows your dignity. You go out a well man in the prime of your life and not a sick man. [At this, Mr Singh straightens appreciably. It obviously touches a chord. His tears stop and he joins in the conversation more equally].

(W7D5:10–11)

Sometimes, the change in a person is so profound that the ward sister actively calls upon a former, different understanding of the patient. When Mr Sykes, a laryngectomy patient, is admitted with recurrent cancer, he is very depressed and silent. Sr Ellis actively has to recall how he was previously.

Sr Ellis: It's less than a year since Mr Sykes came in. And he was a very bright, chatty gentleman. And he's just like a different man. I have to keep reminding myself of that person who came in here. And remember he's the same person.

(Int. 5–2:14–15)

The patients' families also sometimes need to be reminded that the person who is ill is the same person he always has been, even though there may be considerable physical changes after disfiguring surgery. The patient's outward appearance may prompt the family to see someone different. Sr Ellis seeks to help families to understand that it is the person who recovers or dies, not just bits of him. In working with the patient and family, the ward sisters ask them to call on their previous experience in order to gain an understanding of the patient's current pattern.

The ward sisters listen to patients who have had previous surgery. They incorporate the patients' previous experience in their interpretation of recovery. Sr Fraser is giving hand-over report on Mrs Hart, a 48-year-old woman who had ear surgery for a recurring perilymph leak. Sr Fraser explains her unsteadiness on the third post-operative day, 'She says it takes her about two weeks to get back to normal' (W6D5: 17).

As the ward sisters come to know the person's normal pattern, they recognize what is missing as much as what is there – 'If he doesn't crack a joke by the middle of the day, he's having a sad day' (W1D2–2: 6). When inconsistency in a patient's countenance or pattern is noticed, the ward sisters seek to understand it:

Sr Inglis: There's more to Mr Lowe than meets the eye. He looks so worried and so anxious. You go to him and he says he's feeling better and he's not in pain. Something's not right there.

(W9D3: 15)

Such discrepancies are cues for the nurse to seek out their source. Sometimes they ask outright about a normal pattern in relation to this behaviour. 'Do you sleep a lot or are you feeling unwell?' (W9D3: 17). At other times, such discrepancies prompt the nurse to 'keep an eye' on the patient, watching and listening for further changes, a resumption of what is 'normal' or the development of a new pattern.

The ward sisters do not pretend that they know the 'real' person of the patient in any other context but that of being a patient on the ward. They do not claim to know all there is about a person. They recognize that their knowing is in the context of the surgical ward and the surgical experience.

Sr Inglis: I don't believe in the theory that you've got to know every-

> thing about a patient to nurse him well. My husband wouldn't want to tell an 18-year-old all about himself. He'd tell her what he thinks she should know. And I think we have to remember that. Now I don't think a patient has to tell you because you're a nurse. ... If they want to tell you about a problem, I think you should certainly be aware that there might be a problem. And if you could help, help by all means. But I don't think you should delve in and encroach on their private life. Particularly with my patients. Remember they're only here on an average, seven days. ... We've got to be very careful that we don't get patients telling us something they don't really want to tell us.
>
> (Int. 9–3: 52–3)

This quotation reflects a deep understanding of the vulnerability of patients, and of the privileged position of nurses. For nurses are 'involved in the most private aspects of peoples' lives' (Fagin and Diers 1984: 16). Knowing the 'real' person for the ward sisters, means that their knowing arises from and must remain within the context of their nursing practices.

Time is a key component of the context of knowing the patient. The ward sisters amply recognize that they only know the patient for a very short period of time in the person's life span. And almost inevitably it is a time of considerable stress. To get a sense of the patient's history and interpretation of their situation, the ward sisters frequently seek out the person's stories about their illness, their home and family supports and plans for the future. It is these stories that they tell students and junior nurses to listen for, as 'You can learn a lot from your patients that way'. These stories help the nurses to place the illness and hospitalization in the context of the patient's life. It also reminds them that they will only ever know only a small part of the patients' experience of life.

CONCLUDING COMMENTS

This chapter began with a phrase, 'he's better in himself', and a suggestion that this phrase and others reveal the knowledge of the patient embedded in nurses' everyday practices. It is suggested that the way in which the excellent experienced nurses in the study come to know the person of the patients in their care is inextricably tied up with how they practise and experience nursing those patients. The nurses are attuned to the patients and to their ever-changing experiences in the midst of their ongoing work through a process of noticing, understanding and acting.

The way in which these ward sisters practise nursing, and in so doing get to know patients, is characterized by a process akin to dialogue. Even though the dialogue is not always verbal, the nurses are in continual conversation with their own practices, with their own experiences and with patients and their experiences. The ward sisters keep their own practising: what and how they notice, what they understand and how they act, constantly in question.

It would appear that the ward sisters are in the position to get to know patients and their experience of illness because of how they stand with patients and their families, and walk alongside them during this time. From a concernful, involved stance, the ward sisters keep the patient at the very centre of their endeavours. They are committed to knowing them in order to care. Their stance with the patient is always a temporal one, drawing from the past, being in the present and acting toward the future. Time imbues the interpretative process of noticing, understanding and acting. Their interpretation always happens within a particular situation, with its particular temporal, spatial and historical nature and demands. Their knowing is neither timeless nor context-free.

The relational, temporal and contextual nature of experience is revealed in the ward sisters' knowing of the patients. It raises questions about Gadow's contention that illness is 'radically subjective' and has 'like all experience an objective overlay of social meanings, scientific explanations, economic implications' (Gadow 1990: 168). It would appear that the experience of illness can show up in background practices and shared meanings and language.

> One cannot separate life experience from a person's unique interpretation of his or her illness and the ability and desire to get well. Expressions of hope, love, anger, fear, and loss provide the nurse with a lived dialogue, and offer the opportunity for interpretation of events in a way that has particular meaning for the patient. It is from that perspective that the nurse can be in the experience of illness with the patient. ...
>
> (Ryder and Ridley 1990)

It could be argued that it is specious to think that nurses, who are with patients during only a small part of their lifetimes, and perhaps of their illness, could be said to know the person and to understand their experience in any meaningful way. But John Bellany offers a different insight in his portrayal of the ward sister in *A Renaissance*,[2] a series of drawings and paintings which charted the course of his recovery after a liver transplant. The ward sister is present in two or three paintings of the hospitalization period. But what is most intriguing is that it is the ward sister we see in the mirror of his room when he goes home. We see through John Bellany's eyes an important feature of nurses' work. When nurses' practices are smoothly done and accomplished well, they are invisible: their meanings are revealed only in retrospect. It is the presence of the nurse with the patient during the intimate, frequently vulnerable times of illness and recovery that make it possible for nurses and patients to share many of the meanings inherent in the illness experience.

This chapter describes how nurses and patients can travel together during hospitalization for surgery. Nurses are not the only health care professionals who travel with patients and who get to know the patients 'in themselves'. In order to gain other understandings of worlds of illness, there would be merit in exploring the experiences of other health care workers who have the privilege of knowing patients well. Such explorations are needed to help chart the way to better health care.

ACKNOWLEDGEMENT

The author wishes to acknowledge the St Boniface General Hospital Research Foundation and the Committee of Vice-Chancellors and Principals of the United Kingdom for their support of the research which forms the basis of this chapter.

NOTES

1 All names of ward sisters and patients are pseudonyms.
2 An exhibition held at the Scottish National Gallery of Modern Art, 1989.

REFERENCES

Baker, C.A. (1989) 'Recovery: A phenomenon extending beyond discharge', *Scholarly Inquiry for Nursing Practice: An International Journal* 3, 3: 181–94.

Benner, P. (1984) *From Novice to Expert: Excellence and Power in Clinical Nursing Practice*, Menlo Park, California: Addison-Wesley.

Benner, P. and Tanner, C. (1987) 'How expert nurses use intuition', *American Journal of Nursing* (January): 23–31.

Benner, P., Tanner, C., Chesla, K., Gordon, D. and Wros, P. (1991) 'Clinical knowledge: The phenomenology of knowing the patient', paper presented at the Western Institute of Nursing Research Conference, Albuquerque, New Mexico.

Benner, P. and Wrubel, J. (1989) *The Primacy of Caring: Stress and Coping in Health and Illness*, Menlo Park, California: Addison-Wesley.

Bishop, A.H. and Scudder, J.R. (1990) *The Practical, Moral, and Personal Sense of Nursing: A Phenomenological Philosophy of Practice*, Albany, NY: State University of New York Press.

Brown, L. (1986) 'The experience of care: Patient perspectives', *Topics in Clinical Nursing* 8, 2: 56–62.

Carper, B.A. (1978) 'Fundamental patterns of knowing in nursing', *Advances in Nursing Science* 1: 13–23.

Closs, S.J. (1991) *A Nursing Study of Patients' Night-time Pain, Analgesic Provision and Sleep Following Surgery*, Nursing Research Unit, University of Edinburgh, Edinburgh.

Conrad, P. (1987) 'The experience of illness: Recent and new directions', *Research in the Sociology of Health Care* 6: 1–31.

Corbin, J. and Strauss, A. (1985) 'Managing chronic illness at home', *Qualitative Sociology* 8: 224–47.

Dreyfus, H. (1980) 'Holism and hermeneutics', *Review of Metaphysics* 34: 2–23.

Fagin, C. and Diers, D. (1984) 'Nursing as metaphor', *International Nursing Review* 31, 1: 16–17.

Freidson, E. (1986) *Professional Powers: A Study of the Institutionalization of Formal Knowledge*, London and Chicago: University of Chicago Press.

Gadamer, H-G. (1975) *Truth and Method*, London: Sheed and Ward.

Gadow, S. (1990) 'Response to 'Personal knowing: evolving research and practice'', *Scholarly Inquiry for Nursing Practice: An International Journal* 4, 2: 167–70.

Heidegger, M. (1962) *Being and Time*, trans. J. Macquarrie and E. Robinson, Oxford: Basil Blackwell.

Hosang, P. (1991) 'Conversation with author', April, Winnipeg, Canada.

Kesselring, A. (1990) 'The experienced body, when taken-for-grantedness falters: A phenomenological study of living with breast cancer', unpublished Ph.D. dissertation, University of California, San Francisco.

Lathlean, J. (1987) *Job Sharing a Ward Sister's Post*, report of an evaluation commissioned by the Riverside Health Authority, Peterborough: Ashdale Press.

MacLeod, M.L.P. (1990) 'Experience in everyday nursing practice: A study of 'experienced' surgical ward sisters', Ph.D. thesis, University of Edinburgh.

Magee, B. (ed.) (1987) *The Great Philosophers*, London: BBC Books.

Marram Van Servellen, G. (1982) 'The concept of individualized care in nursing practice', *Nursing and Health Care* (November): 482–5.

May, C. (1991) 'Affective neutrality and involvement in nurse-patient relationships: perceptions of appropriate behaviour among nurses in acute medical and surgical wards', *Journal of Advanced Nursing* 16: 552–8.

Meleis, A.I. (1985) *Theoretical Nursing: Development and Progress*, Philadelphia: Lippincott.

Merleau-Ponty, M. (1962) *The Phenomenology of Perception*, trans. C. Smith, London: Routledge & Kegan Paul.

Polanyi, M. (1958) *Personal Knowledge*, rev. edn 1962, London: Routledge & Kegan Paul.

Rabinow, P. and Sullivan, W.M. (1979) *Interpretive Social Science*, Berkeley: University of California Press.

Ricoeur, P. (1979) 'The model of the text: Meaningful action considered as text', in P. Rabinow and W.M. Sullivan (eds) *Interpretive Social Science* (73–101) Berkeley: University of California Press. (First published in Social Research 38, 3, 1971.)

Ryder, R.L. and Ridley, M.G. (1990) *'The place from which the patient comes'*, Journal of Professional Nursing 6, 5: 255.

Sacks, O. (1985) *The Man Who Mistook His Wife for a Hat*, London: Duckworth.

Saxton, M. and Howe, F. (eds) (1988) *With Wings: An Anthology of Literature by Women with Disabilities*, London: Virago Press.

Seers, C.J. (1987) 'Pain, anxiety and recovery in patients undergoing surgery', Ph.D. thesis, King's College, University of London.

Strauss, A., Fagerhaugh S., Suczek B. and Wiener, C. (1985) *Social Organization of Medical Work*, Chicago: University of Chicago Press.

Taylor, C. (1971) 'Interpretation and the sciences of man', *Review of Metaphysics* 25, 1: 1–51. (Also in Taylor, C. (1985) *Philosophy and the Human Sciences. Philosophical Papers* 2, Cambridge: Cambridge University Press.)

Thorne, S.E., and Robinson, C.A. (1988) 'Reciprocal trust in health care relationships', *Journal of Advanced Nursing* 13: 782–9.

Van Manen, M. (1977) 'Linking ways of knowing with ways of being practical', *Curriculum Inquiry* 6, 3: 205–28.

Webb, C. (1986) 'Professional and lay support for hysterectomy patients', Journal of *Advanced Nursing* 11: 167–77.

Wilson-Barnett, J. and Batehup, L. (1988) *Patient Problems: A Research Base for Nursing Care*, London: Scutari Press.

Name index

Subject index